HERBALISM

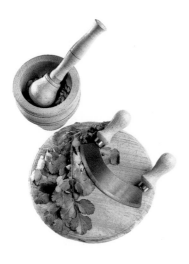

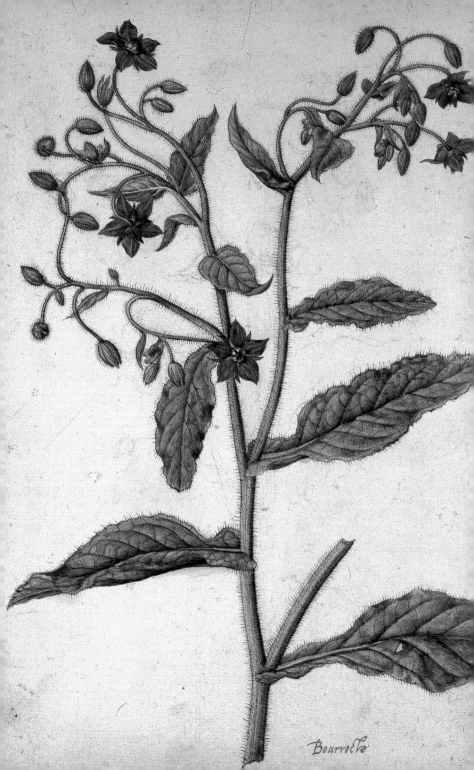

Bourroche

LIVING WISDOM

HERBALISM

FRANK J. LIPP

SERIES CONSULTANT: **PIERS VITEBSKY**

Little, Brown and Company
BOSTON NEW YORK TORONTO LONDON

Contents

First American Edition

Conceived, Edited, and
Designed by
Duncan Baird Publishers
London, England
Editor: Clifford Bishop
Designer: Steve Painter
Picture research: Jan Croot, Liz
Eddison
Commissioned artwork: Jane
Bennett

ISBN 0-316-52750-5

Library of Congress Catalog
Card Number: 95-79151

10 9 8 7 6 5 4 3 2 1

Published simultaneously in
Canada by Little, Brown &
Company (Canada) Limited

Color reproduction by
Colourscan, Singapore
Printed in Singapore

Introduction

Herbs are any plants which have a use, whether as medicines, foods, preservatives, flavourings, cosmetics or scents. As Western technological society has moved further away from using plants in all these roles, so the term "herb" has shrunk in its popular application to a handful of food flavourings and some "alternative" medicines. In this book we return to the original, wider definition. Plants have played an important role in the history of medicine, and some of the world's greatest healing agents have been derived from the plant kingdom. Yet medicinal herbs that were formerly esteemed are now commonly dismissed as placebos. This book examines medicinal plant use within the context of the modern scientific, political and regulatory framework, as well as in traditional cultures across the world.

Perhaps the most extensive investigation of medicinal plants has been in the Chinese, Ayurvedic and Thai medical systems. In each of these traditions, the use of herbs is governed by complex worldviews and explanatory models of the human body and its relationship to the universe. Herbal medicine is the oldest and most widely used form of medicine in the world. The cultural diversity of herbal traditions conceals many common trends that reach back into antiquity. Worldwide, plants are not only foods and medicines, but are also the source of many of the aspirations, myths, symbolic meanings and ritual behaviours of humankind.

Contemporary society is racked by the misuse of plant-derived drugs such as coffee, alcohol, cocaine, heroin and tobacco. Most of these psychotropic, or mood-altering, plants were originally used only in ritual contexts for sacral purposes. Torn from their complex cultural origins, these plants and their derivatives have proven to be a curse to the cultures that have relocated them into a fast-living, restless, consumer-orientated world. Psychotropic plants must be considered in the context of innumerable complex and subtle connections between religious belief systems, ritual and therapeutic practices.

It is important to understand the ways in which plants are beneficial, and to know the safest and most effective ways of preparing them. The adage "prevention is better than cure" is borne out by recent scientific discoveries which underscore the role that plant foods, such as broccoli and garlic, play in preventing cancer and cardiovascular disease. However, many herb-users prefer to emphasize a variety of nonmedical uses, including cosmetics and perfumery. Whatever their purpose, the most satisfying way of obtaining medicinal herbs is to grow them, preserve them and prepare them at home.

WARNING
Plants work as medicines only because they can have a powerful effect upon the human body. In addition, some healing plants look very similar to other, poisonous, plants. Never use a plant unless it is prescribed by a qualified herbalist or unless you are absolutely sure of its botanical identity, its safety and how to use it. The information contained in this book is introductory in nature and is not intended as a substitute for professional knowledge. Neither the publishers nor the author can accept any responsibility for the unsafe use of plants by readers.

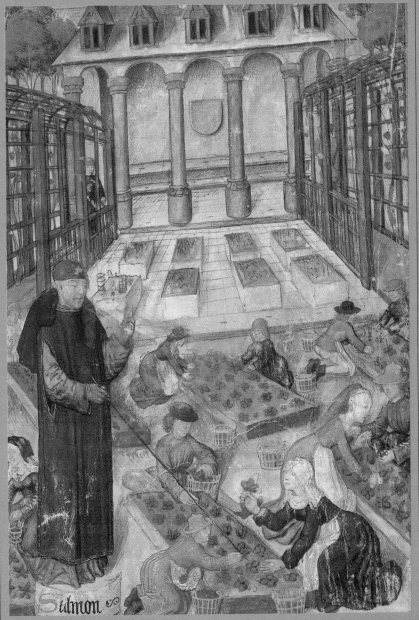

Even as recently as the 17th century, the word "vegetable" was a rarity: people spoke of pot herbs, salad herbs, sweet herbs and simples. This garden of "herbs" was painted in the 15th century.

Plants and People

Plants are the basis upon which all other life depends. Humankind relies, directly or indirectly, upon the plant kingdom for oxygen, fuel, medicines, food and micronutrients, clothing and building materials as well as for many other necessities. Moreover, since prehistory, people have not only drawn upon plants for their material value but have also imputed to the plant world sentiments which are religious, aesthetic, poetic and moral. As indicated by Mendel's hereditary experiments with peas or Pasteur's development of the germ theory of disease using yeast, plants play a significant role in the development of human knowledge.

However, the world's wetlands, island, coastal and desert floras, forests and grasslands are rapidly dwindling before human expansion. Trees are dying because of a disruption of cellular photosynthesis caused by air pollutants, which may affect food plants in the foreseeable future. If the current mass extinction of plant species continues, 25–50 percent of the world's present biodiversity will be extinct in the next generation. These sweeping changes will leave the finite world ecosystem less prepared to adapt to and survive changing conditions, and will ultimately threaten human survival.

To bemoan the disappearance of the rainforests because of the loss of many plant species with potential economic or medicinal properties is only to continue the ethic of nature-as-an-object-of-exploitation. In order to avoid ecological disaster, a profound change of philosophy is required, recognizing the complex unity and kinship of humans, plants and all living things.

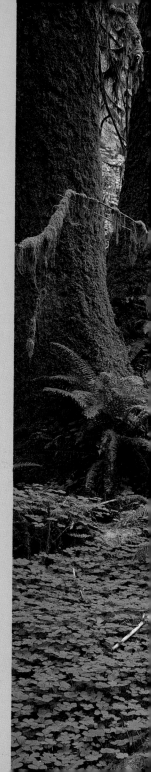

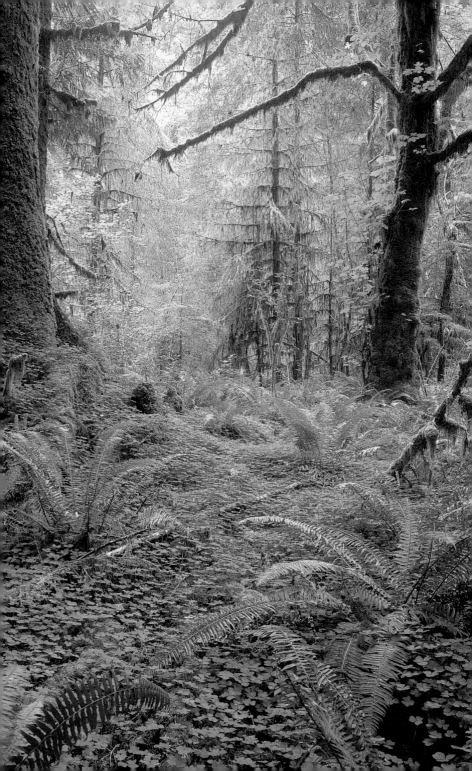

The domain of plant medicines

The comparatively limited concept of a plant "medicine" as a substance that possesses or is reputed to possess curative or remedial properties is restricted to Western society. In many areas of the world the definition is extended to include medicine that makes people fall in love with the user, medicine for winning sales, medicine to appease the ancestors, or anything that is unusual, sacred and imbued with magical power, such as the medicine-shirt of the Plains Native Americans.

"Medicine", according to this conception, involves using the inherent potency of an object to maintain, restore or even upset the balanced harmony of any person, place or thing. There is, moreover, no hard and fast distinction between "medicinal plants" and "food plants", since many plants, such as maize, chilli peppers and sage, are utilized both as food and medicine. Dietary regimes are prescribed for sick or convalescing individuals and certain dietary systems may prevent or – as in the case of a steady diet of "junk" foods – lead to disease and nutrient-deficient behavioural disorders.

Medicinal plants are more than simply objects with useful chemical and symbolic aspects. They are living organisms that are functionally embedded in the cultural fabric of social groups and institutions. They play an integral role in ideas of balance and cosmological order that often reflect sophisticated medical theories of the human body, the symptoms it experiences and their underlying causes.

Many different elements are involved in the complex of ideas and practice that comprises medicinal plant-use. They include a broad network of kin and friends, diverse medical specialists, patient–healer relationships and therapeutic processes. There are specific times at which plants may be gathered, prayers and offerings associated with their collection, modes of preparation and dietary, sexual or other restrictions that can be associated with specific plants. The exact constituents of a medicinal plant-related tradition vary from culture to culture to form a rich and diverse array of medical systems.

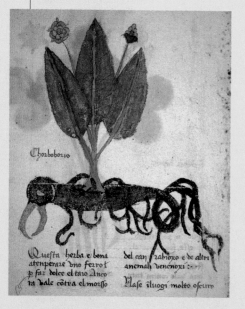

Many herbs have been used historically to treat illnesses that modern Western medicine would consider to be outside the domain of plant cures, or to treat what would not be considered illnesses at all. This illustration from a 14th-century Italian herbal shows a plant labelled Herba corboboris, *which was used to treat anger and the after-effects of surgery.*

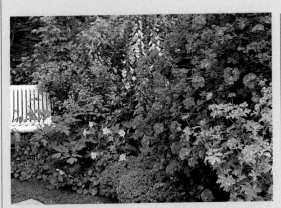

A garden for the blind, filled with aromatic plants. Such gardens can ease depression and prolong the lives of those who use them.

ACTIVATING A CURE

A plant's medicinal potency may lie dormant until the requisite incantation has been pronounced which will define its purpose and direct its action. In order to treat fevers, healers in Zaire go to the sacred section of the woods where the ancestors lie buried, gather the herbs and pray at the moment that the sun's last rays fade away. The ancestral spirits are petitioned to make the fever's heat fade in the same way as the light of the sun.

THE MANDRAKE

No European plant has more beliefs and rituals associated with it – or better reveals the huge variety and range of what can be considered "medicine" – than the mandrake. Because of the resemblance of the forked mandrake root to the human form, it was credited with human and superhuman powers. In pre-industrial Europe, it was dug up near the summer solstice, before sunrise in the last quarter of the moon. The plant throve under gallows and was not easily caught. To keep it still, urine or blood had to be poured on it. Those who ventured to gather it stopped their ears to guard against deafness and insanity from the deathly shrieks which the plant uttered when disturbed. These tales were narrated by collectors to maintain a high price for the roots: a single root in 1690 cost the annual salary of an average artisan.

Mandrake was used in love magic and to secure a favourable judicial decision.

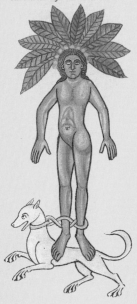

A mandrake-root doll had the power to make its owner invisible. The doll also revealed hidden treasures, but these would only cause misfortune, and eventually bring the doll's owner to an end on the gallows where the plant was first discovered.

Mandrake was used to treat arthritis, ulcers, boils, inflammations, to induce menses, ease delivery and promote animal and human conception. It was also dispensed as an antitoxin for snakebites and an anodyne for wounds, as well as being administered to induce sleep. Containing mandragorine, hyoscyamine and other hallucinogenic tropane alkaloids, mandragora was a potent ingredient in the ointments European witches rubbed on their bodies to enable them to fly.

A mandrake from a 13th-century English herbal.

Therapeutic efficacy of plants

Throughout history medical practitioners have turned to plants and other natural materials to provide them with remedies for disease. Although some of the therapeutic properties that have been attributed to plants are now thought in the West not to be genuine, most medicinal plant therapy is soundly based upon the empirical findings of thousands of years. For example, ancient Egyptians used the fruits and leaves of the bishop's weed (*Ammi majus*) to treat vitiligo, a skin condition characterized by the loss of pigment. A drug (8-methoxypsoralen) has been produced from this plant to treat psoriasis and other skin disorders, in addition to T-cell lymphoma. Claims made in the 18th century that the Indian poke, or pokeroot (*Phytolacca americana*), is effective against cancer were at one time discounted, although the plant has recently been shown to kill cancer in mice.

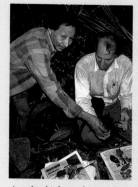

An ethnobiologist learns about the therapeutic uses of local plants from a native of the Amazon forest.

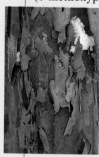

The western yew tree yields a treatment against ovarian cancer.

One-quarter of all medical prescriptions are based on substances that come from plants, or from plant-derived synthetic analogues, and about 80 percent of the world's population – primarily those in developing countries – rely on plant-derived medicine for their health care.

During the last 40 years at least a dozen potent drugs have been derived from flowering plants. They include the *Dioscorea*-derived diosgenin (from which all anti-ovulatory contraceptive agents have been developed), two powerful anti-cancer agents from the African rosy periwinkle (*Catharanthus roseus*), pilocarpine (from South American trees in the citrus family) to treat glaucoma and "dry mouth", and an agent to treat heart failure which is derived from the foxglove (*Digitalis* species). Although discovered accidentally during the course of laboratory observation, two of the major sources for anti-cancer drugs on the market were derived from plants used medicinally by Native Americans: the western yew tree (*Taxus brevifolia*) and the May apple (*Podophyllum peltatum*).

The scientific literature is replete with studies indicating the effectiveness of specific plants against viruses, microbes, inflammation, fungal infections and carcinogenic chemicals. With developments in biotechnology, such as molecular receptor-binding bioassays (procedures which test drugs directly on proteins, rather than living animals) and automated screening facilities, thousands of plant extracts can be tested for a spectrum of diseases daily. In order to keep this highly sophisticated technology in operation, drug companies collect plants and other natural products, such as marine organisms, insects, leech anticoagulants, and spider, snake, and frog venom. Two important results of this chemical prospecting are alkaloids from a Cameroonian rain forest vine and an Australian chestnut tree showing activity against the AIDS virus.

Yet, for the most part, these findings are not followed up, because of the lengthy and expensive procedures involved in testing and developing a drug for regulatory approval. In fact, commercial research investment in plant-derived drugs has been dwindling for much of the 20th century and, at the end of the 1970s, for a time ground to a halt. One reason for this was that after a 20-year, multi-million dollar plant screening effort by researchers for the US National Cancer Institute not a single agent of general use in the treatment of human cancer was identified. However, the tests used a mouse leukaemia cancer as the only screen, whereas cancer comprises some 200 disease types. Currently, Japan, France and many other countries are actively studying and developing plant-derived medicines while the United States is lagging behind.

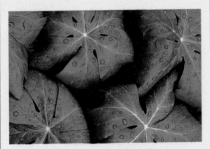

The May apple is used to combat leukaemia, lymphoma and lung and testicular cancer.

SAFETY FACTORS

The therapeutic value of botanical drugs depends upon several factors, including purity, potency and correct dosage. A low dose may be ineffective and the margin of safety between dosages that are correct and fatally excessive, as with digitalis drugs (derived from the foxglove, right), is at times quite small. To achieve the necessary accuracy, crude drug plants must be standardized in terms of growing conditions, harvesting, drying and storage conditions, as well as precise dosage. These standardized procedures are frequently lacking.

Pharmaceutical disparagement of herbal medicines, however, is based on more than scientific criteria. The discovery that a plant grown on a windowsill will prevent an ailment which provides drug companies with a part of their market is an economic threat. The chemical constituents of plants, if published, cannot be patented. In the absence of a profit incentive, drug companies are reluctant to develop plant-based drugs.

However, in many cases the synthetic analogues of plant constituents do not reproduce the biological activity of the natural substance. Some 2 billion dollars are spent annually on herbal medicines and food supplements in Europe and, given the popularity and marketing opportunities, drug companies are buying up smaller herbal medicine companies.

How plants cure

The prevailing scientific view is that all disease is caused on a molecular level. Cholesterol molecules, for example, cause heart disease by forming obstructions in the lining of blood vessels. Similarly, a chemical drug produces its effect by entering a cell through a receptor (a chemical structure on the surface of the cell) that conforms to the shape of the drug molecule, like a lock and key. In contrast, medicinal plants are described by their adherents as working on a higher physiological level (astringents make muscle solids firm; diaphoretics promote perspiration by the skin), which makes them more versatile. A plant that increases the secretion of urine can also be used to treat kidney and bladder ailments or to eliminate body poisons. For example, tannins are compounds that bind with proteins in the skin and mucous membranes and convert them into insoluble, resistant tissues. So plants that are high in tannins, such as bilberry, may be used for a number of ailments, including diarrhoea, wounds, inflamed gums, haemorrhoids and frostbite.

Medicinal plants commonly have several constituents working together catalytically to produce a combined effect which surpasses their individual activity. Taking vitamin C pills is not the same as eating an orange, and there are marked differences between taking a drug, such as caffeine, and using the plant from which the drug is derived. Modes of preparation and ingestion are also important. An anti-cancer alkaloid from the Chinese *Camptotheca acuminata* was discarded during clinical trials because it was toxic to the liver. This was later found to be the result of intravenously administering a substance normally taken orally.

Since the time of Plato it has been recognized that substances with no inherent chemical efficacy are nevertheless useful in eliminating symptoms and

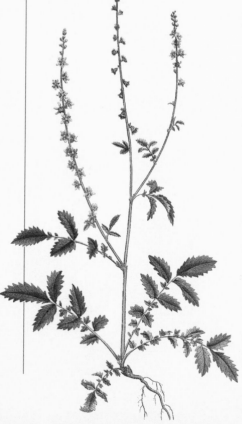

LEFT *Agrimony, from the 19th-century herbal,* Flora Danica, *by Oeder. Although agrimony is primarily a diuretic, its astringency also helps stop urinary bleeding.*

pain. These inert placebos, such as sugar pills or saline injections, are widely given to patients to please or gratify them. It has been estimated that 35–45 percent of all prescriptions are for drugs that by themselves could not affect the conditions for which they are prescribed. People who readily respond to placebos produce more pain-killing morphine-like substances (endorphins) in their body tissues. The effectiveness of the placebo depends on the confidence of the patient in the medications, the powers of suggestion, empathy and charismatic personality of the healer and the dynamic rapport of the doctor–patient relationship.

If attitudes and emotions can affect the onset and course of a disease, then virtually all illnesses can be influenced, positively or negatively, by the mental state of the individual. Feelings of despair in the face of a serious illness, such as AIDS or cancer, can impair the immune system. Emotional stress can also lead to hormonal imbalances, and the patient's will to recover plays a crucial role in any healing process.

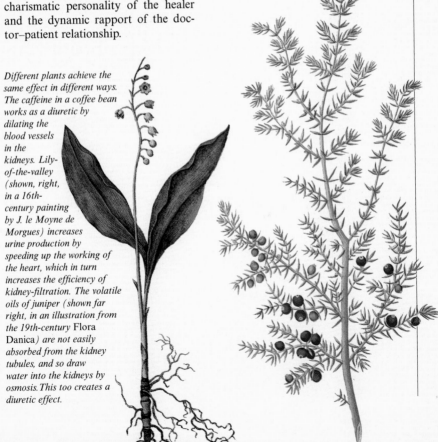

Different plants achieve the same effect in different ways. The caffeine in a coffee bean works as a diuretic by dilating the blood vessels in the kidneys. Lily-of-the-valley (shown, right, in a 16th-century painting by J. le Moyne de Morgues) increases urine production by speeding up the working of the heart, which in turn increases the efficiency of kidney-filtration. The volatile oils of juniper (shown far right, in an illustration from the 19th-century Flora Danica*) are not easily absorbed from the kidney tubules, and so draw water into the kidneys by osmosis. This too creates a diuretic effect.*

Plants and politics

Concern about environmental degradation, the trend to stay green and lead a healthier life, the growing esteem for natural, alternative products and the reaction against what many see as the overspecialized, dehumanized and excessively technological aspects of biomedicine have all revitalized the use of herbal remedies. Yet, although herbal medicines are a thriving multi-million dollar business, the medicinal use of plants is in a subordinate position economically, legally and politically to technologically-based medicine.

Scientific biomedicine is so powerful not because it can refute the ideas behind alternative therapies, or prove those therapies ineffective. Rather, other disciplines and forms of knowledge are marginalized and denied opportunities to compete, either economically or in the realm of debate. Recognition of alternative therapies has been blocked in France, for example, because some 11 percent of the parliamentary deputies are members of the medical profession. However, one in five households in Paris currently uses herbal medicines, as the French, along with many others in the industrialized world, increasingly resort to divergent, pluralistic medical traditions.

Regulatory policies regarding herbal medicines vary from country to country. In France and Britain plant medicines which have a long record of use are considered safe and effective. Germany has a regulatory commission which reviews all plant medicines for approval. In Canada, medicinal plants are reviewed for safety by an expert committee, but are considered to have no proven efficacy and are sold under the category of "folklore medicines". In the United States all drugs must be proven to be both safe and effective. Since this is costly and time-consuming, and herbal medicines are unpatentable, most herbal products are sold in health food stores with no accompanying information regarding properties, dosage, precautions and adverse effects.

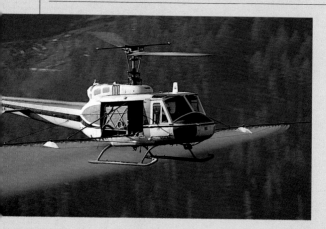

PESTICIDES

There are 3 million severe pesticide poisonings each year, with 220,000 deaths worldwide. Health authorities document the problems arising from herbal medicines and supplements, yet no clinical trials are set to determine the safety of over 100,000 foreign chemicals that are released into the environment annually.

A helicopter sprays for bud worm in Montana, USA.

Among the reasons for official misgivings regarding plant medicines are the unsubstantiated and often extravagant claims made by herbal advocates and the uncritical way in which herbal books are compiled. One popular book, for example, subscribes on average twenty-three different medicinal uses to each plant, with angelica prescribed for cancer, electric shock, tuberculosis and so on.

Plato's description of the Greek word *pharmakon* as meaning "cure" and "poison" suggests the early recognition that many plants simultaneously contain medicinal and potentially toxic substances. Prune juice, taken as a laxative, may produce diarrhoea, and liquorice root, active against gastric ulcers, can in large doses cause heart failure. *Ricinus communis* (castor oil) seeds yield a strong laxative but are highly toxic, and several common medicinal plants including chamomile, marigold and yarrow may produce minor allergic reactions. Advocates of herbal medicines tend to minimize potential dangers, whereas pharmacologists and health authorities emphasize

LIKE TO TREAT LIKE

Homeopathy uses substances that cause the same symptoms as the disease to be cured, in order to stimulate the body's natural defences. These "cures" are only prevented from being poisonous by being diluted down until often no active agent remains in the prescription.

Samuel Hahnemann (1755–1843), the founder of homeopathy.

any harmful effects. Cases of adverse reactions to herbal medicines are rare and often caused by misidentified or incorrect plant mixtures, harmful interaction of the herbal medicine with a prescription drug, poor quality control, or overconsumption and too prolonged a use of a herbal remedy.

Compared with the dangerous side-effects of many pharmaceutical products and the thousands who are killed or maimed by biomedical intervention each year, the risks of herbal medicines are low. The advanced herbal medicines marketed in Europe, for example, are generally safe, although certain imported herbal products distributed by mail or sold in health food stores are sources of concern. One product for asthma was found to contain arsenic, cockroach extract and strychnine.

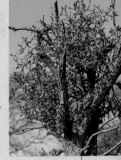

Mistletoe (above), sassafras bark, comfrey, coltsfoot and calamus are among the common plants that contain carcinogenic chemicals.

FRENCH LITIGATION

Maurice Mességué, the famous French herbalist, primarily used external hand- and foot-baths in his practice. Among his patients were Winston Churchill, Cocteau, Utrillo, Ali Khan and King Farouk. He was brought before the French courts by the medical profession twenty-one times for practising without a licence, but won every case.

Disease, medicine and history

The earliest records describing the use of medicinal plants were written by the Assyro-Babylonians and the Egyptians. One of the oldest and most important documents is the Egyptian Ebers papyrus (c.1550BC), which includes more than 700 prescriptions using natural products such as caraway, coriander, garlic, linseed, peppermint, figs, fennel, anise, poppy and castor oil. In ancient Greece there was a guild of rhizomatists or root collectors, who gathered, prepared and sold medicinal plants. Aristotle and Hippocrates developed a theory of the body's primary qualities and balance of fluids, or humours, which determined the use of medicinal plants for 1,500 years.

The Greek botanist and physician, Dioscorides (AD40–90), compiled the first systematic description of 579 plants and their 4,700 medicinal uses

and modes of action. His work, known by the Latin translation *De Materia Medica* (c.65AD), was of central importance to European medicine until the 17th century. Galen (who was born in 131AD) elaborated the properties of the plants described by Dioscorides and further developed the Hippocratic humoural conception of the body.

In hospices and hospitals throughout the Dark Ages, Arab physicians conducted research on medicinal plants collected from India to Spain, and translated the works of Dioscorides and other early botanical writers. At the end of the 11th century, Arab knowledge and practice was introduced into European medicine and remained important until the 16th century. Meanwhile, Christian monks and nuns had since 500AD been establishing cloisters and physic gardens all over Europe, where herbal books were compiled and medicinal plants cultivated and used in infirmaries. Among the most notable were the cloister of the abbot Wilifrid Strabo near Constance, the Benedictine cloisters of St Gallen and Monte Cassino, and that of Hildegard of Bingen, who cared for the sick and described 300 plants and their medicinal uses in her work, *Physica*. Paracelsus (1493–1541), known for his Doctrine of Signatures (see p.45), emphasized the medicinal use of refined chemical substances and ushered in the practice of pharmacy.

Rapid European expansion during the 15th and 16th centuries resulted in

A page from an early 11th-century British copy of De Materia Medica, *which was written in both Latin and Anglo-Saxon.*

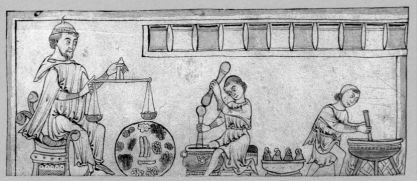

This illustration of an apothecary's workshop from the 12th-century British herbal, De Nomibus Herbraicis, *indicates the growing medieval commercialism in the use of plant medicines.*

the introduction of new medicinal plants, such as ipecacuanha (used as an emetic), cinchona bark (used as quinine to treat malaria and cardiac arrhythmia) and Peru balsam (which was in great demand as a cough remedy and for the external treatment of wounds and scabies). The following centuries witnessed medical botany becoming increasingly separated from and adversarial to academic medicine. Following the coal-tar revolution of the late 19th century, synthetic drugs have increasingly dominated medical practice;

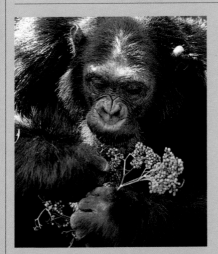

Tanzanian chimps use Aspilia – *which contains a powerful antibiotic – to treat upset stomachs.*

THE PREHISTORY OF PLANT CURES

The use of plants to cure humans is probably as old as the human race itself. Analysis of the pollen of flowers found in a 60,000-year-old Neanderthal grave indicated the presence of marshmallow, yarrow, *Ephedra* – an anti-asthmatic and cardiac stimulant – and four other plants that may have been used for medicinal purposes by the local Iraqi population. Ice-age art is primarily concerned with fauna, but floral bouquets, wild grasses and branches with leaves appear occasionally in cave paintings and on mammoth ivory.

Some folk traditions describe medicinal plants as gifts from the gods, others hold that the use of certain plants was learned by observing animals. For example, swallows are said to apply the juice of the greater celandine to the cloudy eyes of their young, tortoises eat marjoram after being bitten by snakes and weasels heal themselves by eating rue flowers.

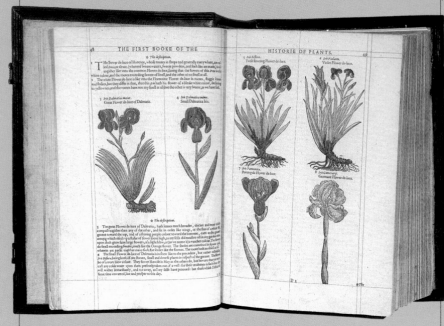

Although valuable medical compendia, or leechbooks, were written throughout the Middle Ages, it was the printing of Dioscorides' herbal in 1478 that inspired a florescence of herbal works by, among others, Fuchs, Brunfels, Gerard (whose illustrations of Fleurs-de-luce *are shown above), Bock and Culpeper. Hand-copied herbals had been too rare and expensive to reach the general public, but popular medical editions created an overlapping zone between patrician and popular medicine.*

nevertheless, medicinal plants are still widely used today.

Although many diseases, such as pyorrhoea and arthritis, have always existed, the patterns of mortality caused by different diseases have changed dramatically throughout history. It is important to understand this process in order to evaluate the medicinal plants used under different historical and cultural conditions.

Hunting and gathering populations are generally healthy and fit, with well developed coordination and vision. The !Kung and San, of Africa, for example, are able to see four of the moons of Jupiter with the naked eye. Viral infections are infrequent and limited to those, like herpes simplex and chicken pox, marked by latency or recurrence. Low population density and a scattered, mobile existence cannot support measles and other viral infections that are characterized by eventual recovery and immunity. Skeletal material from hunting and gathering groups displays less disease and/or nutritional stress than skeletal samples that come from, for example, ancient agriculturists of the New World. Cancer, cardiovascular and chronic diseases are infrequent, and mortality is predominantly a result of venomous organisms, wild beasts, trauma, warfare and fighting. This is reflected in the uses that hunters and gatherers have found for medicinal plants. The Andamese Islanders, for example, have only 20 herbal remedies limited to colds, fever, malaria, sepsis, injuries and bone fractures, toothache, body pain, swellings and gastrointesti-nal and gynaecological disorders.

The range of traditional medicinal plants in an agricultural population is more complex and reflects marked eco-logical and cultural changes. The agri-culturist Shuar of the Ecuadorian Amazon possess 245 medicinal plants, 104 of which are for gastrointestinal disorders and 98 for skin ailments, reflecting the impact of tropical rainfor-est conditions on health. Similarly, of 99 plant species used medicinally by the warlike agricultural population of New

PATTERNS OF ILLNESS AND PATTERNS OF CURE

Changes in the use of herbal remedies are clear indicators of evolving disease patterns but often occur rapidly and are difficult to detect. However, during a recent 40-year period, medicinal plant use among rural Mexicans in Texas shifted from remedies for work-related traumas and infections to herbal treat-ments for cancer, hyperten-sion and diabetes: changes in emphasis that all indicate a rural-to-urban shift in life style. At the same time, there was no change in the herbal treatments for the common cold, gastrointestinal disor-ders and skin irritations.

Plant therapy, although equipped to treat a formidable number of diseases, was developed under pre-industrial conditions and is in fact largely unable to deal with cancer and the other diseases of civilization which were

little known and almost non-existent until recently. Although the use of plants, animals and mineral matter constitute a major component of all traditional medical systems, they are combined with blood-letting, cauterization, diet, enemas, fumigation, heat, music and incantation, as well as a variety of exorcisms via mediums or shamans.

Sweat-baths were used for colds, malaria, rheumatism and other diseases from Ireland across Eurasia and into Central America. The outlawing of the native sweat-house in 16th-century Mexico by the Spaniards contributed greatly to Indian mortality, since *syphilis trepenoma* and other pathogenic organisms perish under high temperatures.

The Florentine codex of 1570, showing a range of healing methods used in Central America, including sweating and bone-setting.

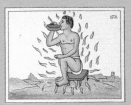

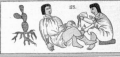

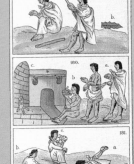

Guinea, 53 percent are used for wounds and aches, with the rest being employed for first aid, intestinal problems, skin conditions, fevers, natal care and tonics.

The domestication of plants and animals resulted in settled communities and increased population density, permitting the rapid transmission of infectious viral, bacterial and protozoan micro-organisms, as well as constant reinfection. Contaminated water supplies, inadequate disposal of human excreta and sewage, houseflies and the use of human offal as fertilizer brought cholera and many other viral and bacterial diseases. Domestic animals

Despite the prevalence of high technology biomedicine in the 20th century, Victorian evaporating dishes are still used in Britain to produce herbal extracts.

served as hosts for agents of typhoid fever, anthrax and tuberculosis. Malaria and schistosomiasis (carried by mosquitoes and water-snails, respectively) spread because of irrigation, while deforestation was responsible for the spread of yellow fever, dengue and scrub typhus. Nutritional disorders such as beriberi, sprue and kwashiorkor appeared when humans began living on diets consisting largely of grains.

Epidemics of infectious diseases intensified with the growth of pre-industrial cities and the proliferation of flocks, crops and humans. The decimation of both hunting and agricultural populations in America and elsewhere by measles, whooping cough, influenza and scarlet fever epidemics indicates that these populations were not exposed to the relevant pathogens prior to European colonization. Similarly, Europeans were affected by diseases, such as yellow fever in Africa, to which local inhabitants had acquired considerable genetic resistance.

JUNK FOODS

Hypertension, heart disease, strokes and diabetes among Australian Aborigines, Pacific Islanders and other peoples are strongly linked to a rapid changeover from traditional foods to fatty, sugary, overly refined fast and packaged foods. The Tohono O'odham, Pima and Cocopa of the Arizona desert, for example, have extremely high rates of obesity and diabetes, caused recently by the abandonment of tepary beans, mesquite pods, prickly pear cactus and other soluble fibre- and carbohydrate-rich foods. Groups such as the Mormons, who restrict their fat and meat intake, suffer less from colon and breast cancer than the surrounding population.

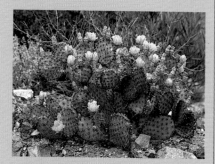

Carbohydrates contained in cacti and other desert foods are digested and absorbed slowly, without producing a rapid increase in blood sugar and stress on the pancreas.

THE LEGACY OF INDUSTRIALIZATION

During the Industrial Revolution of the 19th century, urbanization and rapid population growth in Europe were marked by frequent and severe outbreaks of infectious diseases. The transmission of tuberculosis, diphtheria, smallpox, typhoid fever and other diseases was exacerbated by intense squalor, poverty, overcrowding, long hours of work and malnutrition.

Great reliance was placed upon herbal remedies that were sold in town markets by country people, since physicians did not minister to working class families too poor to pay for treatment. The decline in mortality toward the end of the century was probably more a consequence of improvements in sanitation, diet and general standards of living rather than vaccination and other medical advances. Today the leading causes of death in industrialized countries are cardiovascular diseases and cancer, caused by synthetic chemicals, radiation, industrial pollutants such as lead and pesticides, over-consumption of high-fat diets, tobacco, alcohol and inadequate exercise. Despite billions of dollars spent on research, the overall incidence of cancer increased by 18 percent between 1973 and 1990. Although the immediate cause of cancer is tumour-producing genes,

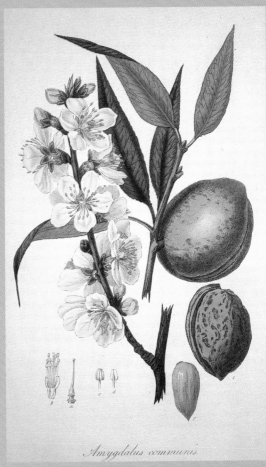

Amygdalus communis.

An almond, taken from a 19th-century medical botanical text. By the 19th century, the Linnaean system of plant classification had helped to establish botany as a distinct science, and the fanciful herbal illustrations of the past were replaced by more precise, taxonomically useful paintings.

such as *p16*, the ultimate causes are embedded in our industrial environment. Many sophisticated and costly biomedical services have been developed largely to treat diseases which are a direct consequence of contemporary life and urban, industrial development.

Western and traditional medicines

Attempts to give precise definitions of "traditional medicine" have always given rise to argument, since the phrase encompasses everything from !Kung shamanic healing in Namibia to the Ayurvedic and other, highly formalized, systems of India (see p.77). Although a global definition of traditional medicine may not be possible, certain key features can be detected.

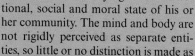

Traditional medicine considers the self to be intimately linked with the social, moral and religious order. The restoration of an individual's health is achieved by purifying the emotional, social and moral state of his or her community. The mind and body are not rigidly perceived as separate entities, so little or no distinction is made as

A government health worker in New Guinea applies Western rather than traditional methods.

to whether it is the mind or the body that is affected by an illness, or whether the illness has been caused by psychological or organic processes. The body is not seen as an independent entity, separate from other people, strong emotions, spirits and natural forces.

In the allopathic approach which has come to dominate Western medicine, diseases are treated with specific drugs or procedures whose physical effect is the opposite of the illness (this contrasts with homeopathy, see p.17). According to this worldview, all diseases have biological causes and are classified according to the body tissue, organ or system involved. The body is perceived as a complex machine which can be described by the use of scientific categories and explanations. A highly sophisticated medical technology has arisen from this approach, which has historically emphasized procedures aimed at cutting, probing and investigating. The theoretical basis of allopathy means that, in most orthodox

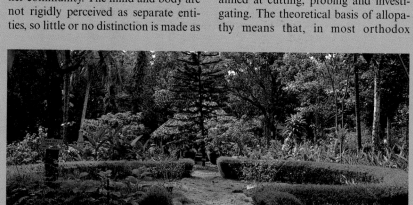

The herb garden of an Ayurvedic clinic in Kerala. Although Ayurveda is considered to be traditional, its procedures and classifications are as complex and systematic as those of Western medicine.

MAGIC AND MEDICINE

The concepts and practices of non-Western and pre-industrial medical systems are commonly described by Western commentators in terms of a dichotomy between the magico-religious and the rational. All phenomena relating to illness and curing in a culture are classified as being either empirical or magical, either rational or mystical.

However, these categorical abstractions – which are derived from Western thought – are foreign to the worldview of peoples for whom religion and medicine have not split off from one another and are closely interwoven with all other aspects of the culture. In the Fipa language, for example, there are no terms corresponding to our words for "medicine" and "magic", since the language itself does not distinguish between forms of knowledge, and therefore does not differentiate between these ways of knowing.

Illness touches upon fundamental aspects of the human condition which are experienced in non-Western societies as disturbances in the relations that encompass an individual. The projection of Western categories on to the experiences and ideas of other peoples fails to do justice to the complexity of their own therapeutic

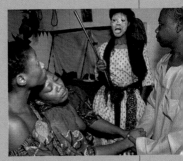

Haitian voodoo priests heal – and harm – through the use of spirits and possession.

realities. The division of the world into the mystical and the rational is itself a pre-conceived view of reality, which cannot ultimately be considered authoritative.

Western medicine, the body and mind are treated as though they are distinct. Indeed, healing is perceived as being dependent upon the separateness of the mind and body. However, the placebo effect (see p.15) shows that there is still a psychological element in the practice of Western medicine, whatever its theoretical background.

By contrast, traditional medicine defines good health as a state of equilibrium. The curing process attempts to restore balance and harmony between physical, spiritual and social functions. The doctor and patient share a common worldview and relationships between them are informal, close and based on day-to-day interaction. Traditional healers are minimally organized, part-time specialists with an authority based upon charisma and reputation. In Western medicine, doctor–patient relationships tend to be impersonal and couched in a technical language. Western hospitals are hierarchical, with organized, rule-governed staff, and authority is established by credentials, licences and scientific titles. These features reflect the evolution of scientific medicine in highly populated urban societies, characterized by many casual or contractual interactions.

Traditional medicine is more often found in societies with enduring relationships focused upon the family, kin and community. An entire community will frequently be involved in traditional therapies, contributing materials, labour and prayers. Medical instruments and drugs are hand-made, grown or found in nature, and curing is carried out at home or at a shrine.

Herbal Lexicon

People who read herbals – ancient and modern – are often taken aback by the great number of diseases that any one plant is claimed to be capable of alleviating. Yet most of the plants mentioned in herbals have a long history of medicinal use, and the diseases that have been treated by them are therefore quite extensive. This lexicon describes the uses and the cultural and historical backgrounds of forty common European medicinal plants, which have been selected on the basis of their popularity, usefulness and safety.

The uses of medicinal plants change over time, and many of the diseases mentioned here are evocative of the widespread ailments of earlier periods. Plants, long discarded as being ineffective, can be reinstated and become fashionable for a while, only to be replaced by other cures. Several of the plants included have overlapping medicinal, nutritional and cosmetic functions, and are readily available in the form of teas, tinctures, pills, creams and bath additives.

Although these plants are of European provenance, many are distributed and used throughout the world. The harvesting and collection times given are for temperate Europe and North America, where the average last frost is at the end of April and the average first frost is at the end of October. Readers in other parts of the world should adjust the recommended times accordingly.

A physician weighing ingredients for a herbal cure, from a 12th-century German Herbarium *by Apuleius Platonicus.*

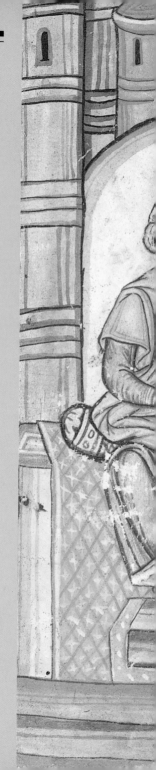

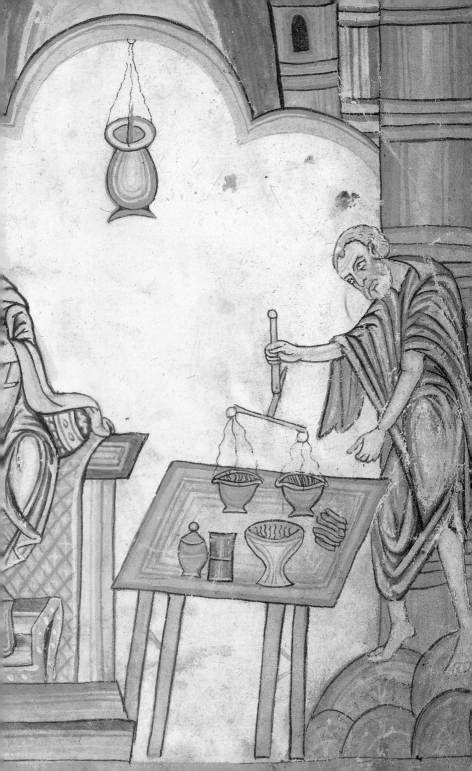

Yarrow *Achillea millefolium*

Dried herb

Yarrow, or milfoil, is an aromatic perennial with woolly stems up to 3ft (1m) in height, which prefers light, sandy soil and grows in fields, open woodlands and along roadsides. The flowering stems are collected in June and July. As an aromatic bitter, yarrow stimulates the appetite and a tea mixture composed of yarrow, chamomile and peppermint is recommended for gastrointestinal and gall problems. Yarrow also promotes sweating and a hot yarrow tea is a folk medicine for fever, colds and influenza. A high content of calcium and other substances which stimulate kidney activity make the tea especially appropriate for spring and autumn tonics.

The essential oil and flavonoids of yarrow have anti-inflammatory, disinfectant and antispasmodic properties. Yarrow staunches external and internal bleeding of the intestines, kidney, nose, lungs and uterus,

giving rise to the origin of another of its traditional names, "thousand seal". Wounds are tended with a boiled extract of the plant and the treatment of internal bleeding is supported with yarrow-baths.

As a fresh juice extract, yarrow is said to stimulate the general metabolism, improve the circulation of the blood and raise the body's ability to resist disease. Yarrow is specific for the treatment of a circulatory disorder in women (parametropathia spastica), which is characterized by spasmodic pain in the small of the back and abdomen, hypermenorrhoea and pain in the breasts prior to menstruation.

The mixed, fresh extracts of yarrow and watercress are used as a spring tonic for chronic mucous secretions of the lungs and urinary tract. The fresh juice of the plant may also be applied in a poultice to ulcers and boils. However, some people are allergic to yarrow: if skin rashes occur, treatment should be discontinued.

WAR AND DIVINATION

The ancient Chinese threw yarrow stalks when consulting the I Ching, their book of divination, and until the 19th century the plant was used in rural Europe to divine a future mate and to test a lover's fidelity. The yarrow was plucked from the grave of a young individual of the opposite sex and put

under the pillow after a formula had been recited. The future mate then appeared in a dream. The magical uses of yarrow survived for centuries in Europe alongside its medicinal uses: these same rural communities used the chewed plant to cure festering wounds.

The scientific name for yarrow derives from Achilles,

the Greek warrior-surgeon, who learned of the curative properties of this "soldier's wort" from the centaur Chiron. In the *Iliad*, Achilles sprinkles roots of yarrow to heal the wounds of his friend, Petroclus. During medieval tournaments and battles, and in the American Civil War, yarrow was used as a surgical dressing to stem the flow of blood.

Lady's mantle *Alchemilla vulgaris*

Lady's mantle grows in bushes, moist fields and on the borders of forests. The leaves are collected in June and July, when the morning dew and the plant's active exudations have dried. The plant takes its scientific name from the alchemists who collected the liquid that is exuded on the leaves for their magical experiments. The common name reflects the resemblance of the folded, mantle-like leaves to the scalloped edges of the Virgin Mary's mantle, which protects all of Christendom.

The plant has styptic and astringent properties and is active against acute, non-specific diarrhoea, enteritis and other gastrointestinal disorders. A cupful of hot water is poured over a spoonful of the macerated leaves, left to stand for about 10–15 minutes, and taken two to three times daily.

Lady's mantle tea has been used to treat menopausal disorders, prevent excessive menstrual bleeding and as a douche to treat leucorrhoea, a whitish vaginal discharge that occurs in young girls. As a wash, it is used for oozing eczema, purulent wounds, inflamed eyes and as a gargle for sore throats and inflamed mucous membranes.

Burdock *Arctium lappa*

An aromatic, biennial plant growing to 3ft (1m) in height, burdock grows on waste ground, by roadsides and alongside streams. The roots are collected in the autumn or early spring and air dried. Burdock contains iron, niacin, vitamin C and inulin, which is beneficial for the lungs, liver and gall.

Burdock is diuretic and diaphoretic and, as a tea, is used for colds, coughs and stomach disorders. It has been an essential ingredient in traditional blood-cleansing teas. Two teaspoons of root are allowed to stand in a 1 pint (50cl) cold water infusion for 5 hours, boiled, strained and taken three times a day.

The plant is antibiotic, pain-reducing and fungicidal, and consistent use is prescribed for a wide variety of skin conditions. A syrup prepared from the root or the fresh leaves is used as a wash or poultice for skin irritations, burns, wounds, gout, boils, measles, acne, ringworm, herpes, eczema and mange. A decoction of burdock and nettle roots – a quarter ounce (10g) each in half a pint (25cl) of water – together with a little vinegar is a stimulating hair tonic, and a preparation of burdock root and olive or sesame oil is recommended for itchy, scaly scalp conditions.

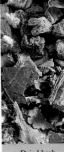

Dried herb
Dried root

Onion and garlic *Allium sativum* and *Allium cepa*

Like the ancient Babylonians, Austrian farmers use onions to "fix the fates" on New Year's Eve. They fill twelve onion sheaths with salt, and the ensuing months of the year will be dry or wet, according to whether the salt in the corresponding peel remains dry or forms a fluid.

The onion was a basic food and medicine in Greece, and the Romans ascribed twenty-seven medicinal uses to it. In 16th-century Europe onions were used to treat upset stomachs, burns and wounds, to expel worms and to aid sleep. During World War II, onion paste was applied to severe burns in order to prevent infection.

Onions stimulate the appetite, assist digestion and alleviate coughs, sore throats and congested lungs caused by colds. An old cure for colds is to macerate an onion and mix it with 3 spoonfuls of honey. This is cooked for several minutes in 1.5fl oz (12.5cl) of water and left to set. Made fresh each day, 1–2 teaspoonfuls are taken three to four times a day.

The garlic plant, native to central Asia, is used in China to treat high blood pressure, and in India for abdominal tumours. The Jews used garlic cloves both to treat melancholy and to expel worms, while the Copts prescribed a garlic cure to cleanse the intestines and clear the head.

The Roman historian Pliny describes 61 disorders for which garlic was employed, including asthma, sprains, toothache and venomous bites. In European herbal medicine, garlic is

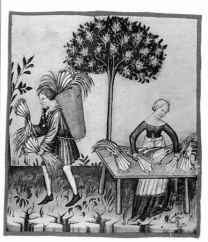

People selling alliums, *from the 14th-century Italian* Tacuinum Sanitatis, *by Ibn Botlân.*

In ancient Egypt, the pyramid-builders received their pay in onions. In Pharaonic medicine, onions were prescribed to prevent, among other complaints, a wasting disease of the limbs, which the Egyptians called "blood eating". Onions found widespread use in mummification and as a form of snake repellent. As such, onions were anathema to the harvest goddess Renenutet (right), in her manifestation as a snake goddess. However, other gods and goddesses held the onion in high esteem. The Egyptians regarded the onion bulb as a symbol of the universe and sacred to the mother-goddess, Isis. The consecutive onion skins about the centre corresponded to the concentric, layered spheres of Egyptian cosmology.

used to improve digestion and blood circulation, to expel wind, for stomach cramps, gall bladder infections, acute infections of the gastrointestinal system, arteriosclerosis and high blood pressure.

Millions of people today use garlic not to treat specific diseases but rather to enhance the body's immune response and general state of well-being. Garlic counters blood conditions that foster hardening of the arteries, heart attacks and strokes. It contains alicin and other biochemicals which reduce low density cholesterol and the oxidation of other potentially harmful blood fats, as well as promoting the regression of fatty deposits in the blood vessels and dissolving arteriosclerotic blockages in coronary arteries. Garlic also cleanses the blood by hindering the clumping of blood platelets, helping to dissolve existing blood clots and increasing both arterial dilation and capillary blood flow.

Diets rich in garlic are associated with low rates of cancer. Garlic contains organic sulphur compounds which prevent carcinogenic chemicals from converting normal cells into cancer cells, and may inhibit the growth of malignant cells. The constituents of garlic break down dangerous nitrosamines (in the stomach, colon and rectum) and other chemicals which can cause cancers of the breast and oesophagus. Garlic compounds also protect cells against damage by heavy metals.

Garlic is not always beneficial. In large amounts it may produce anaemia, stomach inflammations and ulcers, and suppression of testicular function. For those who wish to avoid bad breath, deodorized garlic extracts provide the same benefits as fresh garlic.

EVIL SPIRITS

Garlic has long been a means of protection from evil spirits and magic. The Romans used garlic to conjure away mischievous spirits of the dead and Greek soldiers carried it in small bags or in their caps to ward off sorcery and misfortune.

In Estonia, infants were supplied with garlic in amulets at baptism and underneath their pillows to fend off demons and witches.

Garlic wreaths were hung up in Romanian stables to protect the animals from contagious diseases and thunderstorms. Romanians also placed garlic cloves in the harvest grains as a defence against witches, and in the mouths of corpses thought to be vampires.

In Cuba, Switzerland and eastern Europe garlic was hung around the necks of children as sympathetic medicine for the evil eye, jaundice and other illnesses.

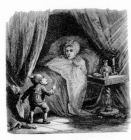

Swedish bridegrooms wore garlic as a defence against envious elves of the sort depicted in this 19th-century Scandinavian illustration.

Marshmallow *Althaea officinalis*

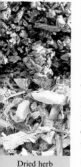

Dried herb
Dried root

Marshmallows, also known as mallards, sweet weeds and wymotes, grow to 5ft (1.5m) in height, and are commonly found in coastal salt marshes and on saline soils in damp meadows. The roots and leaves are collected in the spring or autumn after the flowering period, and are quickly dried to prevent fungal infestation. The botanical name, *Althaea*, is probably derived from the Greek word *altho*, "to heal". The Greeks used marshmallow to treat stings, ulcers and wounds, and the Romans inherited this reverence for the herb. A dish of marshmallow was a great Roman delicacy, and Pliny believed that whoever took a spoonful of mallow in the morning "shall that day be free from all diseases that may come to him".

Arab physicians used marshmallow to treat inflammations, and the Christian Emperor Charlemagne (742–814AD) ruled that the plant should be cultivated in gardens throughout his empire. Because it had been thought by the Greeks to allay heat, marshmallow was used in the Middle Ages to circumvent the ordeal of holding a red-hot iron, which was used to test a person's innocence. By covering the hands with a thick coat of marshmallow sap, fleabane seeds and eggwhite, the suspected person's hands were easily shielded from the heat.

A high content of sweet, viscous mucilage gives the root its pain-soothing, lubricating and anti-inflammatory properties. Marshmallow syrup has long been used for hoarseness, sore throats, coughs brought on by colds, bronchitis and inflammation of the digestive and urinary tracts. Applied externally as a warm poultice, it soothes pain and irritations caused by burns and inflammation of the eye. Marshmallow-mash brushed on linen is good for boils.

Mucilage-containing herbal remedies should not be boiled or cooked. The macerated root of marshmallow is set in cold water overnight and the solution slightly warmed, strained and a tablespoon swallowed. A leaf-tea is prepared by pouring a cup of hot water over 2 teaspoons of the leaves and allowing them to set for 10 minutes. The unsweetened tea is used in a compress on wounds, as a gargle or is drunk for gastrointestinal ailments.

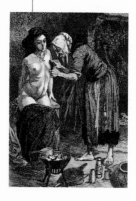

A salve made from the leaves of marshmallow was widely used to rub the body of anyone affected by witchcraft, as shown in Martin van Mael's 16th-century illustration of a village wise woman tending to her client, taken from Michelet's La Sorcière.

Bearberry *Arctostaphylos uva-ursi*

Dried leaves

This heather-like plant prefers a cool climate, and sandy or rocky areas with acid soil. It grows on moors, in coniferous woods and on mountain ridges. The scarlet fruits of the bearberry are meally and tasteless. They are avoided by cattle, but are favoured by grouse. The leaves are collected in late summer and autumn, and should be dried with moderate heat.

The first mention of bearberry as a herbal remedy is in 13th-century Wales, among the so-called Physicians of Myddfai, from where it spread to the rest of Europe. It was described by the botanist Clusius in 1601, but did not find its way officially into the *London Pharmacopoeia* until 1788. Because of its high tannin content, it was not only used medicinally, but also to dye leather and wool.

Bearberry is now considered useful primarily as a disinfectant for a variety of bladder and kidney conditions and, in particular, for acute inflammation of the urinary bladder which commonly appear after colds. A tea made from the leaves or the berries cooked to a thick syrup is a highly recommended remedy for chronic inflammation of the urethra. It is also used to treat renal haematuria, uterine ulcers, retention of urine, chronic cystic catarrh, kidney inflammation and gravel and kidney stones.

Bearberry tea strengthens, contracts and increases the firmness of the membranes of the urinary organs. The tannin content released when the leaves are boiled is good for treating diarrhoea but may lead to nausea and vomiting. In general, care must be taken when using bearberry, as overconsumption, or preparation with boiling water, may lead to stomach disorders and poisoning.

Two of the main chemical constituents in bearberry leaves are arbutin and methylarbutin. These metabolize to form the main bladder and kidney antiseptic, hydrochinone, but only do so in non-acidic urine, so that a tea made with sodium bicarbonate should be included as part of the treatment, in order to alkalize the urine.

Preparing the leaves in a cold water infusion for 12–24 hours releases the active chemicals but not the bitter tannins. A half pint (25cl) of cold water is poured on to 1–2 teaspoons of leaves and stirred occasionally as it steeps, before finally being strained. The infusion is warmed slightly and taken two to three times a day for at least 3 days. Bearberry has been used in this way to treat chronic leucorrhoea, excessive menstruation and vaginal infections.

Bearberry was also known to the pre-European Native Americans, who used it for sprains, swellings, poison-ivy rash and as a tobacco admixture. Early travellers on the Pacific northwest coast reported that smoking bearberry had a narcotic effect.

Horseradish *Armoracia rusticana*

Dried root

Horseradish is widely cultivated, and may also be found growing wild along roadsides, although it prefers marshy or moist areas. For medicinal purposes, the root is gathered in late autumn and covered with dry sand or earth in a cool, dark, frost-free area, or in the refrigerator. Care should be taken in grating the intensely acrid and pungent root, which has a similar effect to chopping onions. The plant contains an antibiotic mustard oil that is active in the treatment of kidney and urinary tract infections, chronic bronchitis and other infected or congested chest conditions. Having a high content of vitamin C, potassium, sulphur and calcium, horseradish has been used in treating both scurvy and anaemia.

For coughs caused by colds, a teaspoonful of equal amounts of grated horseradish and honey or sugar can be taken three times a day. A horseradish mash may be taken for metabolic disturbances, sluggish bowel movements and to expel worms in children.

Horseradish contains sinigrin which stimulates capillary blood flow beneath the skin, and freshly grated horseradish spread on a cloth and applied as a compress has been used for arthritis, rheumatism and sciatica. A compress made of the freshly grated and mashed root has also been a home remedy for inflamed nerves, neuralgia, headaches, muscular aches, toothache, dizziness, fainting and choking. The grated roots can be steeped or boiled in milk, or decocted with alcohol or vinegar, to make a skin-cleansing lotion. The juice of the fresh leaves soothes cuts, burns and chilblains.

As a food or spice, horseradish stimulates the appetite and aids digestion, but should be taken sparingly. Strong doses irritate the kidneys and gastrointestinal system, and may cause vomiting or bloody urine. Care is also to be given in the use of horseradish poultices, which should be applied for no more than 10 minutes at a time.

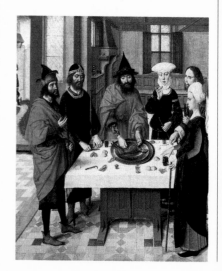

Horseradish is native to eastern and southeastern Europe. The taste, momentarily sweet but quickly turning bitingly sharp, made its adoption in the rest of Europe a gradual one. Horseradish is one of the five bitter herbs that are ritually taken on the Jewish Passover feast, as shown in this altarpiece panel from St Peter's, Leuven, painted by Dirck Bouts (1415–75). The horseradish grinder was a familiar character in Jewish communities.

Wormwood *Artemisia absinthium*

Wormwood prefers to grow in warm areas near the sea, but it is also commonly found on stream banks, waste ground and roadsides. The flowering plant is collected when it starts to bloom, in May and June, and is dried in the open. The botanical name of the plant is taken from the Greek deity of childbirth, Artemis. It was used by the ancient Greeks and Romans to induce regular menstruation as well as in secret incantations to call forth spirits of the dead and demons of the underworld. In pre-Christian Europe wormwood was used for burning corpses and later to decorate Christian biers. It was also planted on graves, hence its symbolic connotation of melancholy.

Wormwood stimulates the appetite and is used as a spice for roast goose

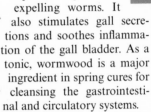

Dried herb

and other fatty dishes. It is effective in the treatment of bad digestion, flatulence and other stomach ailments and, as the common name implies, is good for expelling worms. It also stimulates gall secretions and soothes inflammation of the gall bladder. As a tonic, wormwood is a major ingredient in spring cures for cleansing the gastrointestinal and circulatory systems.

To prepare wormwood tea, 1 tablespoon of the herb is cooked in a cup of water and left to set for 10 minutes. A cup of the warm tea is taken two or three times a day after meals. Wormwood should not be taken by pregnant women. Overconsumption or prolonged use leads to inflammation of the kidneys, nervousness, muscle cramps, headaches, dizziness and blurred vision.

Wormwood is a powerful stimulant, antiseptic and fever-cure, which has been used to treat cystitis, nervous dyspepsia, constipation, jaundice and dropsy. As a compress or salve, it is applied to bruises, sprains, local irritations and arthritic or rheumatic joints.

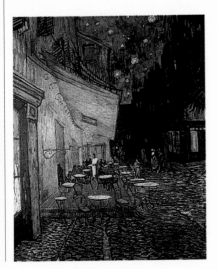

Wormwood was used to impart a bitterness to beer before hops were employed for this purpose, and it is used today in vermouth. It was also the active ingredient in absinthe, a favourite liqueur of many 19th-century writers and artists, such as Rimbaud, Verlaine and Van Gogh, who painted this view of the café at Arles in 1888. Absinthe has been illegal in France since 1915, because it is habit-forming and with repeated use causes permanent damage to the nervous system.

White birch *Betula pendula and Betula pubescens*

Tree silhouette

The birches are an important part of the northern forests of both the Old and New Worlds. With the recession of the Pleistocene glaciers, the birch, with the ash, was the first tree to repopulate the Eurasian continent, and all Indoeuropean languages have a related word for this tree.

Both the major European species, the silver or warty birch, *Betula pendula*, and the downy birch, *Betula pubescens*, are used medicinally. The silver birch is a larger tree, with a silvery white bark and young twigs covered with wart-like resin glands, and grows in drier areas. The downy birch has a denser, furry coat on the young shoots and prefers moist woods, moors and swamps.

The sap is collected in the spring, whereas the leaves and bark may be collected in the spring and autumn, before being dried at room temperature.

Birch-leaf tea has diaphoretic, deworming and astringent properties, and is an excellent diuretic which increases the production of urine without overstimulating the kidneys. Hence, it is effective in dispelling urinary gravel and stones, and treating inflammatory, bacterial diseases marked by spasms or cramps. Birch leaves are an essential ingredient in tea mixtures for kidney ailments, bladder inflammations, cystic catarrh, metabolic illnesses, dropsy and seasonal tonics for gout and rheumatism.

Birch tea – or birch sap – may also be used as a scalp wash to discourage dandruff and hair loss. The sugary sap, rich in vitamin C, is brewed to make a tonic beer. It is also used to treat scurvy and skin eruptions. The tea is prepared by pouring a cup of boiling water over 2 teaspoonfuls of the leaves and straining after 10 minutes. The leaves may be steeped until the water cools, or longer (up to 2 hours), but they should not at any time be simmered or boiled. The warm tea is taken three times a day, preferably unsweetened.

The liquid obtained by boiling the bark is used as an analgesic to bathe stubborn sores and wounds, or as a hot poultice, and the leaves, bark and catkins can all be applied to open wounds, burns and skin irritations. The aromatic birch-tar oil, containing the aspirin-like methyl salicylate which is effective against rheumatism, is used to make oil of wintergreen and medicated soaps for sores and boils.

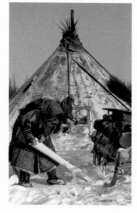

Birches are characterized by a fibrous outer bark that readily peels off in paperlike sheets. This Sakha (Yakut) woman from Siberia is peeling bark from a birch bough in order to use it as toilet paper.

THE SYMBOL AND THE SCOURGE

The fasces, the emblem of Roman magistracy, were made of birch and later the birch rod became the schoolmaster's sceptre of authority and wand with which to control recalcitrant boys. The birch tree is sacred to Thor, the Germanic god of thunder, and embodies the return of spring and its fertilizing forces. In medieval Germany, district councils assembled in groves of birch. A tonic wine, made from the spring sap, was taken for debility, impotence and consumption. When cattle were first driven out to spring pasture, they were ritually struck with consecrated birch rods in order to ensure their health and fertility.

The birch tree was revered by the Finno-Ugrians and other peoples of northern Eurasia. In the Finnish epic, *Kalevala*, Väinämöinen cuts down a forest except for a single birch, and in the Finnish marriage ceremony the couple ritually light a fire made of birchwood. Birch branches are used in Finnish sweat-bath rituals, and to scourge the body in Russian and Finnish baths in order to promote perspiration. In Estonian and Lithuanian songs venerating the birch, people were exhorted to use the bounty of the tree but to spare the heaven-ascending treetop. Special, very old trees were the residence of a birch elf, and among the Sakha (Yakut) of Siberia the

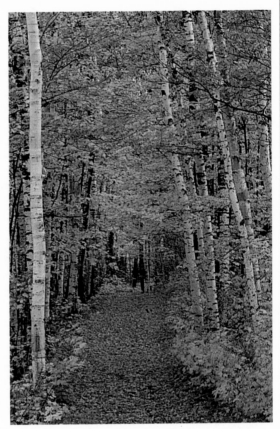

A grove of silver birches. Until quite recently in parts of Europe birch trees were planted in front of houses as protection against lightning and cattle stalls were smoked with the leaves to drive away bewitched vermin. On the evening before Walpurgis Night (1 May), small birch trees were planted and birch sprigs put on barn doors and manure piles to drive away witches.

birch was the doorway for a beautiful, beneficent earth-spirit. The Saami or Lapp woodcutter had to inform the' birch that he was planning to fell it in order to give the spirits living inside time to move, and certain birches were considered so sacred that they were not allowed to be cut down. In traditional Saami medicine, the bark and leaves are used to treat wounds, burns, rashes, in moxibustion (herb-burning cures) and as a spring tonic.

Oats *Avena sativa*

Oats are among the earliest grains to have been domesticated in western Asia and Europe. Oat groats – kernels with their husks removed – and sprouts contain amino acids, minerals, beta carotene and vitamins B_2, K and E, and are high in zinc content. Taken as a soup, porridge, beverage or cereal, oats make an easily digested food which is especially suitable for children. A diet of oatmeal is recommended for diabetics, and to ease inflammation of the mucous lining of the stomach, as well as stomach ulcers, chronic diarrhoea and constipation. An oatmeal poultice helps soothe allergic skin conditions, while a finely ground refrigerated oatmeal face pack is an excellent skin cleanser and conditioner.

Oat tea or extract can be mixed with brier hip (*Rosa canina*) to ease kidney ailments. When used on its own it is a cure for liver ailments and dysentery, as well as insomnia, colds of the throat and larynx, fever, loss of appetite and nervous exhaustion.

The boiled extract of oat-straw also strengthens the nervous system, and is ideal for convalescing individuals who have been weakened by an illness. However, oat straw is more commonly used in baths to open skin pores and to treat rheumatism, abdominal, kidney and bladder ailments, kidney stones and gout. Approximately 4oz (100g) of macerated oat plants are boiled in 6 pints (3 litres) of water for 20 minutes, after which the liquid is strained and poured into a warm, full bath. A simple footbath can be prepared by boiling about 3–5 handfuls of oat-straw in a kettle for half an hour. Feet that are persistently cold, or suffer from hard skin, gout, corns, blisters and ingrown, putrid toenails should be soaked in the decoction at a temperature of 26°C (79°F) for 25 minutes.

Oat tincture is a homeopathic remedy containing a sedative, avenine, which is used by insomniacs and anyone suffering from stress or overwork. Too much consumption of oat derivatives may cause headaches and, as a general cure, uncooked oat flakes, mixed with fruit, honey and nuts, should only be taken in moderate amounts.

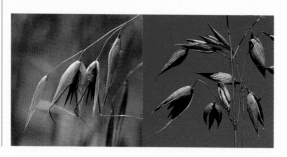

Wild oats (far left) probably originated in western Europe as weeds growing among early strains of barley. They are similar to cultivated oats (left) and in many parts of the world both species may be harvested together for animal feed. Red oats are a heat tolerant variety, widespread in warmer climates.

Marigold *Calendula officinalis*

Marigolds are commonly grown as ornamental flowers, but also occur on waste ground and railway embankments. The blossoms should be collected in dry weather during the summer months and quickly dried at room temperature in an airy place.

A moist, hot compress or dressing saturated with marigold tea is used to heal inflammation of the skin, wounds, ulcers, sprains or dislocations. As a wash, marigold tea is also applied to sore eyes. Taken internally, it has mild diuretic, antispasmodic and diaphoretic properties, and has been used as a general remedy for fevers, stomach ulcers, nausea and nervous conditions.

Dried flower

For gall ailments a cup of the tea is taken two to three times a day, and a cup of the tea may be taken daily from 1 week before menstruation to ease menstrual pain.

A salve, which is rubbed on painful joints and muscles or on the abdomen for stomach aches, is prepared by mixing equal amounts of the crushed leaves with goat butter. A soothing face cream can be prepared with the flower essence, while a strong infusion of the petals tones blemished skin and makes a softening hair rinse for redheads.

Fresh or dried, the petals are a substitute for saffron (and were used as such by the ancient Egyptians), and impart a delicate flavour to rice, soups and stews. The crushed petals and chopped leaves make a tasty addition to salads, and the dried petals are used for buns and baked sweets.

FLOWERS OF THE SUN

The ancient Greeks used marigolds for decoration at their festivals and made them into garlands for their heroes. According to one legend, Caltha, a Greek maiden who had fallen in love with Apollo the sun-god, would remain in the fields all night just to get first sight of his flashing eye. Consumed by her love she wasted away and died, and where she had long stood appeared the marigold, coloured like the sun. In another legend four wood nymphs who had fallen in love with Apollo quarrelled out of jealousy, so the sun-god's sister Artemis turned them into marigolds.

Because their florets resemble rays of glory, marigolds were consecrated to the Virgin Mary. In Elizabethan England, women wore marigold garlands to banquets and bridals, and marigold baskets were sent by gentlemen to the maidens they admired. Marigolds even came to be used as an ingredient in English and Serbian love magic.

Indian marigolds are called "herbs of the sun". They are sacred to the goddess Mahadevi and are worn as garlands at her festival.

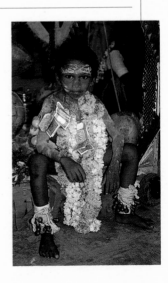

Shepherd's purse *Capsella bursa-pastoris*

Dried seed pods

Shepherd's purse is a small, annual, evergreen plant with a rosette of slightly hairy leaves at its base, arrow-shaped stem leaves, clusters of small, white, inconspicuous flowers at the top, and triangular seed pods (resembling old-fashioned purses). It is a common weed found in gardens, fields, waste ground, and along roadsides. The whole plant, excluding the root, should be collected in the spring and summer, then bundled and dried in a shady place. The peppery young leaves can be used in spring salads or cooked with vegetables.

Although originally a native of the Mediterranean, shepherd's purse is distributed today throughout the world. The plant was used medicinally by the Greeks and Romans to cure hernias, pustules and wounds. It was also used to induce abortions, expel gall and, when applied in the form of an enema, for sciatica. It was believed that, in order to be effective, the plants had to be picked with only one hand. In medieval Europe, in order to stimulate teething in children, the dried pods were sewn in a red linen patch and hung around the infant's neck. After all the teeth had appeared, the amulet was thrown into running water.

Shepherd's purse contains vitamin K – which promotes the clotting of blood – in addition to a blood-staunching peptide. The fresh juice or an infusion of the plant is effective in treating heavy menstrual bleeding, and a ball of cotton saturated with the juice and inserted into the nostrils helps stop nose bleeds. The plant or its juice may be used as a compress on cuts and wounds. However, its blood-staunching effectiveness is inconsistent because of the variable presence of the active principle. It has even been suggested that menstrual disorders are not alleviated by shepherd's purse, but by a fungus which parasitizes it.

Shepherd's purse tea improves the circulation by regulating the working of weakened hearts – especially in the elderly – regardless of whether blood pressure is high or low. The tea is prepared by pouring a cup of boiling water over 1–2 teaspoonfuls of the dried herb. After 10 minutes, the liquid is strained. One or 2 cold cupfuls are taken daily.

Shepherd's purse has diuretic and stimulant properties. It has been used in remedies for catarrh, liver and gall ailments, diarrhoea, stomach ulcers, diabetes, haemorrhoids, bleeding of the uterus, haemorrhages and ulcers of the bladder and ureter.

*The tea made from shepherd's purse is a spring tonic and, taken as a gargle and rinse, is used as a mouth and throat disinfectant. When prepared with horsetail (*Equisetum arvense*), the tea has been used as a remedy for colds, gout and rheumatism.*

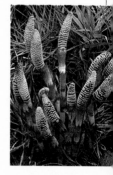

Caraway *Carum carvi*

Caraway is extensively cultivated, and can also be found growing in meadows and on railway embankments. The seeds are collected late in the summer, but great care should be taken because of the plant's resemblance to several of its poisonous relatives.

In medieval Europe the roots were boiled and eaten, and the young leaves added to soups and salads. Caraway potions were used in love magic to cure fickleness in lovers. Caraway tea has also been used to promote menstruation, alleviate menstrual cramps, ease labour pains and to stimulate milk secretion in nursing mothers.

For indigestion and flatulence, 3 drops of caraway oil on sugar may be taken once a day, a handful of the seeds chewed or a tea prepared. A mixture of equal parts anise, caraway and fennel seeds may be cooked in milk, as a remedy for halitosis, gassy indigestion, coughs and mucus due to colds.

Caraway soup is a traditional remedy for stomach aches and dizziness caused by constipation. Cooked in wine, caraway expels worms and eases urinary ailments and haemorrhoids in the elderly. For gastrointestinal conditions, some seeds are put in a bottle of gin or brandy, and placed in the sun for 2 weeks. A teaspoonful of the liquor is taken daily with 5 drops of caraway oil. For respiratory ailments the oil, mixed with a fatty oil, can also be rubbed on the body. Caraway sachets, warmed on a hotplate, ease rheumatic pain, toothache and headaches.

The pungent, aromatic seeds are used in breads and cakes, to season stews and other foods and as a flavouring in Dutch liqueurs. Their aroma increases with age, and the essential oils are used in making soaps and scented sachets.

Seeds

Caraway stimulates the appetite. The seeds are a remedy for indigestion, chronic flatulence, dyspepsia, and flatulent colic in infants. In Elizabethan England, a bowl of caraway seeds was customarily served with apples, and caraway-seed cake was traditionally offered to farmhands upon completion of spring sowing.

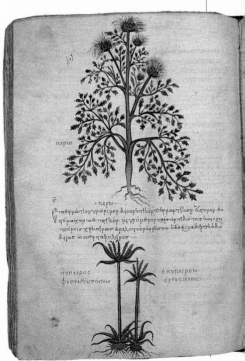

Centaury *Centaurium erythraea*

Dried herb

The European centaury is a shrubby annual which occurs in chalky soil, moist meadows and sunny, wooded areas. The stems and flowers are collected when the plant is in flower from July to September, hung up in bundles to dry quickly, and then wrapped in heavy paper.

Centaury is a bitter tonic that has fever-reducing and deworming properties. It stimulates digestive activity and has been used to treat heartburn, chronic stomach catarrh and stomach weaknesses following acute illnesses. It is particularly effective against digestive ailments arising from insufficient or disturbed secretions of glandular juices. However, different plants should be used for stomach ailments that have been caused by high acidity or irritated stomach nerves.

Centaury stimulates the flow of gall secretions, cleanses the liver and kidney and has been used to treat gall stones, sluggish or obstructed livers, and jaundice. The glycoside bitters (derived from simple sugars) contained in the plant improve circulatory system activity. Centaury tea, taken over a period of time, is recommended for anaemia, circulatory disturbances, blood deficiencies and irregular menstruation.

Having a soothing effect on the nervous system, centaury is also beneficial in cases of depression, psychosomatic conditions due to overstrained nerves, and is specific for curing the eating disorder, anorexia nervosa. The tea is prepared as an infusion of cold water over 2–4 hours and taken in the morning and before retiring, or before meals. It can also be applied to the face to treat freckles and blemishes.

THE CENTAUR'S HERB

Centaury takes its Latin name from the centaur Chiron, who had knowledge of all sciences, especially herbal medicine. In his cave on Mt Pelion, he instructed many young heroes and sons of the gods, including Asclepios, Heracles, Jason and Achilles. Chiron used centaury to cure himself of a wound accidentally received from an arrow that had been poisoned with the blood of a hydra, and some modern herbalists still treat wounds, small ulcers and skin eruptions with centaury.

Like many other reddish-flowering plants, centaury has anti-demonic properties, and was worn as a wreath in pre-industrial Europe as protection against witches and evil spirits. Going to a crossroad on Walpurgis night (1 May) wearing a centaury-wreath enabled one to see the witches flying to the sabbat. The plant was also strewn on the hearth as a protection against thunderstorms.

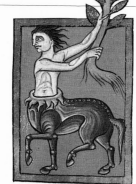

Centaury, from a 12th-century English version of Platonicus's Herbarium.

Chamomile *Chamaemelum nobile* and *Matricaria recutita*

Chamomile is one of the world's most popular healing plants, included in the pharmacopoeia of twenty-six countries, with 4,000 tons produced annually. The preferred type for medicinal purposes is the wild or German chamomile (*Matricaria recutita*). The flower heads are collected three to five days after flowering (they were traditionally collected on or before St John's Day so as to prevent witches urinating on them).

Chamomile's chemical constituents have anti-inflammatory, antiseptic, antispasmodic, antiflatulent and sedative properties. Taken internally, chamomile relaxes smooth muscle and is effective in treating inflammations and irritations of the gastrointestinal lining, uterus, anal and vaginal areas. Taken externally it is considered to heal haemorrhoids, ulcers, burns, severe wounds and skin infections. One chemical constituent, alpha-bisabolol, is used in the treatment of ulcers induced

Dried herb

by alcohol or burns.

For feverish colds, flu and throat infections, a sweat-bath is prepared by pouring 2 pints (1 litre) of boiling water over a handful of the flowers and inhaling the steam for up to 10 minutes. Chamomile teas (which should not be prepared under great heat or steeped more than 10 minutes) and baths have long been household remedies for childhood discomforts, including teething pains, earache, hyperactivity and sleep disorders.

Use of the plant's essential blue oil increases the number of heart contractions and dilates the main blood vessels of the brain. Its sedative properties are used for menstrual pain and cramps, neuralgia and tension headaches, although chamomile may actually cause vertigo and nervousness when used in large doses to expel worms.

OTHER CHAMOMILES

The annual wild or German chamomile is culturally related to the garden or Roman chamomile, *Chamaemelum nobile*. The Roman chamomile is commonly used to flavour Spanish sherry. It can also be used to lighten fair hair or in facial saunas, and may be added to bath preparations, creams, soaps and skin lotions for regenerating tissue and cleansing sensitive, greasy complexions.

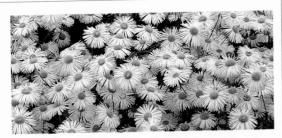

Dyer's chamomile, *Anthemis tinctoria*, has a longer stem than German chamomile. Its yellow flowers can be boiled to give a powerful golden-brown dye.

The Roman chamomile is a perennial, smaller than the German chamomile, with a stronger fragrance. It has similar medicinal properties but is considered less effective.

Chicory *Cichorium intybus*

Dried root

The daisy-like flowers of chicory (or succory) are blue, or more rarely pink or white, and open only in sunshine. The flower heads are gathered in July, but the roots are collected in rainy weather in the late autumn, chopped up and dried in an airy room.

In pre-industrial Europe, the white-flowered chicory was placed under expectant women to assist childbirth, while the bitter, milky juice of the root was used to treat the sore breasts of nursing mothers. For inflammations and cramps of the stomach, the boiled leaves and flowers make an effective remedy, wrapped up in cloth and applied as a compress two to three times daily. A wash of the herb is recommended for sore, tired or inflamed eyes, and an infusion of the flowers and leaves may be applied to the face at night for skin blemishes and soreness caused by the sun.

To prepare chicory tea, 1 cup of cold water is poured on a teaspoonful of the root or flower and leaves, cooked for 2–3 minutes and then strained. Larger amounts may be prepared by cooking 0.7oz (20g) of the root with 6fl oz (18cl) of water for 5 minutes. For stomach ailments a cup is taken before breakfast and in the evening. For liver and gall disturbances chicory is usually taken with chamomile, peppermint and centaury or with peppermint as a seasonal cure. Chicory also acts as a bitter tonic, diuretic and laxative, and has been used as a household remedy for worms, kidney stones, rheumatism, jaundice and nervous conditions.

The young, basal leaves, which are collected before the plant flowers, are cooked as greens or blanched and used in salads. The roots may be steamed or boiled and seasoned with butter, fruit and spices. During Napoleon's blockade of many of Europe's ports, chicory became a popular substitute for coffee and today is added to coffee to balance its flavour and counteract its acidity.

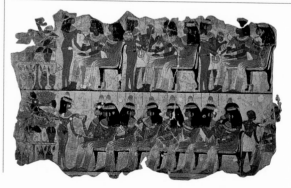

EGYPTIAN ADDITIVE

The Egyptians, and later the Arabs, made great use of chicory leaves in salads. In Pharaonic times chicory juice was added to rose oil and vinegar to treat headaches and was taken with wine to relieve liver and bladder ailments, as is shown in this wall painting of a banquet, from Thebes *c.*1400BC.

Eyebright *Euphrasia rostkoviana*

Eyebright is a small semiparasitic annual which feeds on grass without damaging it. Eyebright prefers sandy or chalky soils, grows in meadows, heaths and sunny woods, and is often found in the mountains and near the sea. The plant, except for the root, is collected at the beginning of the flowering period in June. It is bundled, hung to dry in a shady, airy place and kept in tightly closed containers to prevent spoilage. Plants from alpine environments are considered to be especially potent.

Eyebright has astringent and tonic properties, and is the pre-eminent herbal eye medication. It is used in treating sore, tired eyes and weak vision caused by over-straining while reading and writing. It is beneficial for light-sensitive eyes, styes, colds of the eye, watering eyes and discharges due to allergic reactions. Eyebright is especially recommended for blepharitis (inflammation of the eyelids) and conjunctivitis (inflammation of the connective tissue with mucoid, purulent discharge). Drops of the freshly pressed juice or infusion are dropped on to a small linen cloth, which is fastened upon the eyes with a string until dry. To make the infusion, 2 teaspoonfuls of the powdered herb are boiled with a cupful of cold water, steeped for 2 minutes, strained and some salt added.

Dried herb

A teaspoonful of the pulverized herb or tea should be taken three times a day to supplement external use. In treating eye ailments, eyebright is often prepared in tea mixtures with chamomile, fennel or goldenseal. An eyebright lotion is widely sold commercially to accentuate the beauty and brightness of the eyes.

Eyebright has other uses in herbal medicine, and has found favour as a tonic bitter to aid digestion. It has also been used to alleviate hoarseness, aches and nasal congestion resulting from coughs and colds.

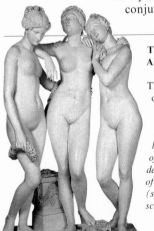

THE IMPORTANCE OF APPEARANCES

The 16th-century Doctrine of Signatures held that the internal powers of a plant

Eyebright improves the beauty as well as the health of the eye. Its Latin name derives from Euphrosyne, one of the Graces of Greek myth (seen here in a 19th-century sculpture by Jean Pradier).

were implied by its external shapes and attributes. The dark pupil-like spot on the corolla, purple veins and yellow flecks of eyebright, similar to a bloodshot eye, designated the plant as a cure for eye ailments. However, although eyebright is indeed a powerful eye medication, the Doctrine of Signatures itself was not accepted by the best herbalists of the time.

Fennel *Foeniculum vulgare*

Seeds

Fennel has been an important culinary and medicinal herb for over 2,000 years. In early Greece, the participants in the Attic mysteries wore wreaths of the herb and athletes ate the seeds as a health food and to control their weight. The Romans ascribed twenty-two medicinal uses to fennel, one of which – the treatment of eye ailments – is also found in Coptic medical prescriptions. The uses of fennel for eye diseases – and a number of related medicinal traditions – have remarkable historical continuity: its eye-healing properties are cited by Hildegard of Bingen in the 12th century and by present-day herbalists.

The Romans especially liked fennel, and cookbooks giving their favourite recipes for the plant are still extant. An early compilation of cooking recipes was assembled by Marcus Gabius Apicius (died AD40), a wealthy Roman who, as his funds dwindled, and fearing he would starve, spent all his money on a final feast and drank a cup of poisoned wine after dinner. In Roman households fennel shoots were cooked as vegetables and the raw stalks added to salads. The seeds were placed under loaves of bread before baking. Roman soldiers and gladiators ate fennel with their meals to increase their fighting strength and courage. The wreaths worn by victors after combat in the arena were made of fennel. The plants were also strewn across the pathway of Roman newly-weds.

The Frankish Emperor Charlemagne the Great ordered fennel to be grown on all royal farms, and from medieval cloister gardens fennel spread into peasant gardens, where it was valued for its ability to satisfy cravings of hunger on Lenten fast days.

Mild and gently calming, fennel makes an excellent tea for treating coughs, flatulence, abdominal cramps and colic in infants and children. Having expectorant, antispasmodic and anti-inflammatory properties, fennel has been used to treat hoarseness, catarrh, halitosis, asthma, headaches, dizziness, depression and delayed menstruation. It also aids milk production in nursing mothers.

As a spice, it is served in salads, soups, sauces, cabbage dishes and with soft cheeses. Fennel stimulates the digestion and cuts the taste of eels, mackerel and other oily species of fish. In Provence, France, fish are grilled over dried fennel stalks to give them added flavour. Fennel is also used as an antidote to snake-bites, an insect repellent and a cosmetic facial. It adds a sharp pungency to potpourris, soaps and shampoos.

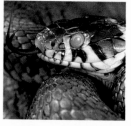

The Romans claimed to have discovered fennel's use as an eye cure by observing snakes who, after shedding their skins, rubbed against fennel plants to improve their eyesight. A snake's eyes are milky, and apparently blind, when it sheds its skin, and clear afterward.

SEASONAL MAGIC

At the ancient Phoenician
midsummer festival to invoke
rainfall, fennel was ritually
planted in clay pots around the
image of the god, Adonis.
The rapid sprouting of the
seeds and subsequent
withering of the sprouts in
the heat was symbolic of the
death and resurrection of
the ephemeral Adonis. The
festival, termed Adonia,
ended with the casting of
the pots containing the
dead fennel and other
plants, along with images
of the deity, into the sea or
a nearby freshwater spring.

In medieval Europe
fennel-wreaths were hung
above doorways on
midsummer day to keep
witches away and, in the
Pyrenees, they were
fastened on rooftops for
protection against evil
magic. In the 16th century,
the *benandante* or good
witches of northern Italy
battled with the diabolical
witches at night, armed
with bundles of fennel
stalks. These battles were
fought by the *benandante*
in an altered state of
consciousness four times a
year in order to protect
the fertility of the fields and to
ensure abundant harvests.

Today, fennel is an important
ingredient in the sacred elixir
used in the initiation ceremony of
the widespread Afro-Cuban religious
cult called Santeria.

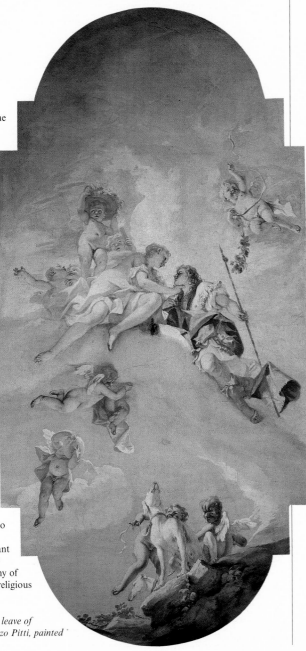

*The goddess Venus taking her leave of
Adonis, from Florence's Palazzo Pitti, painted
by Carlo Ricci in 1708.*

Yellow gentian *Gentiana lutea*

Dried root

Gentian root is effective in treating feeble, sluggish digestion, flatulence and stomach cramps caused by the deficient secretion of gastric juices. It stimulates the appetite and tonifies the digestive system. Used externally, a decoction of the root is applied in a poultice for abscesses and boils. Termed a simple bitter, since it contains little tannin and aromatic oil, the slowly dried, fermented and distilled root has long been an important ingredient in the bitter aperitifs and the brandies of alpine Europe. Known as *Enzianschnaps*, it is a time-honoured folk remedy for fatigue, hunger, aches and pains, and shivering caused by over-exposure to the elements. The cocktail ingredient angostura bitter, which is basically a gentian tincture, may be used medicinally.

Said to stimulate muscles and nerves, gentian tincture is a favourite tonic for travellers, individuals with weak nerves and the elderly. Gentian bitters increase the white blood cell count and are used to treat secondary anaemia. Chewing on the root at intervals during the day is recommended for abating the craving for tobacco, but gentian is not advisable for pregnant women or for those with nervous conditions, high blood pressure and irritated or ulcerous stomachs.

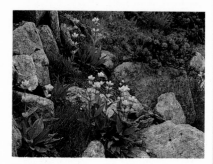

Gentian likes calcium-rich soil, and is found in the meadows and pastures of alpine Europe and Asia. It grows to 3ft (1m) in height but is much smaller at higher elevations. The flowers appear only after several years of growth. Once a troublesome weed for the farmers of the Alps and Pyrenees, it is currently a protected species. Introduced by the Spaniards, gentian is now common in the Andes, where it is used to treat diabetes, nervous disorders and rashes.

PLAGUE CURE

Yellow gentian bears the name of the Illyrian king and herbalist, Gentius who, in the 2nd century BC, recommended it as a protection against the plague. Through the writings of Dioscorides and Galen, the plant was later adopted by the herbalists of medieval Europe. In the 11th century AD, a pestilent disease was afflicting the subjects of the Hungarian king Ladislaus. After praying for divine guidance, he shot an arrow into the air which was found to have pierced a gentian root. The remedy was tried and, according to the account, was instrumental in halting the pestilence. Although this may appear somewhat fanciful, it should be noted that gentiopicrin, a glucoside derived from the plant, is presently used to treat malaria.

Hop *Humulus lupulus*

Native to Europe, Asia and North America, hops are cultivated in all temperate regions and occur wild in moist thickets, along forests, rivers and fences. The hop vine is a perennial climbing to 20ft (6m) and higher. The Frankish king Pepin the Little instituted hop gardens in the 8th century, and in the 12th century hops were introduced into Dutch breweries. The ripened female cones or strobili clarify and impart a bitter flavour to beer and ale, and also prevent bacterial growth in the beer and wort. Hops – which are members of the hemp family (*Cannabaceae*) – were once deemed dangerous because it was noticed that harvesters fell asleep while gathering them.

A tea made from the catkins or leaves is primarily used to treat loss of appetite, mild depression, anxiety and overstimulated nervous conditions. Hops also overcome sleeplessness caused by nervous conditions. (A small pillow stuffed with dried hops was used to cure George III's insomnia in England in 1787.) Hop-derived preparations have also been used to reduce the pulse frequency in nervous tachycardia and to treat war psychosis.

Dried herb

With its diuretic, tonic, diaphoretic, stomachic and sedative properties, the plant has had wide applications in herbal medicine. Boiled in goat's milk, hops were used for scabies, scurvy, herpes and to expel worms. They were made into a salve to ease pain and dissipate boils. The volatile oil is still used to impart a pleasing scent to astringent skin lotions.

Hops also stimulate the glands and muscles of the stomach and remove urinary acid deposits. A salad of the young shoots can be taken as a purgative and to clean the blood. The stems are rich in fibre and the young tops are prepared like asparagus, especially in Belgium.

Hops act upon the reproductive system and have been used to abate painful priapism (permanent erection) and to stimulate menstruation. Native North Americans used hops for many of the same ailments as Europeans.

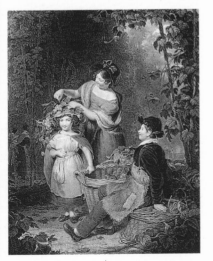

An 18th-century Flemish engraving of hop pickers taking a break from their work.

St John's wort *Hypericum perforatum*

Dried herb

St John's wort is a shrubby perennial growing to 3ft (1m) in height. The five-petalled, bright, golden-yellow flowers occur in branched clusters and have yellow threads in the middle, which yield a blood red juice when bruised. The small, black oil glands on the leaves and flowers have a distinctive odour and bitter taste. St John's wort prefers dry, gravelly or chalky soil and grows in sunny meadows, open woods, shady banks and along hedges and roadsides. The plant spreads vigorously from short runners and produces as many as 30,000 seeds per plant in a single season. The seeds are easily carried by the wind, and have been seen growing in the steeples of old churches. Originally a native of Europe and western Asia, it presently thrives in all temperate zones. Early colonists introduced the plant into North America, but found the Native Americans already using various related *Hypericum* species in much the same manner as they did.

St John's wort has perhaps more medicinal uses than any other plant. Current research is focused on its antibacterial, antibiotic, anti-inflammatory, antidepressive and antiviral properties. Hypericin, a chemical constituent found in the plant, is effective in reducing retroviral HIV reproduction. Because it contains compounds that act as monamine-oxidase (enzyme) inhibitors, St John's wort is

UNIVERSAL PROTECTION

On St John's Eve or Day (24 June) great bonfire festivals were celebrated throughout medieval Europe. Wearing wreaths made of St John's wort the people danced and cast the plant into the fires to ensure an abundant harvest and to protect their cattle from sorcery-induced disease. After the fires were out, the wreaths were thrown on to roofs to protect the houses from lightning, conflagrations and evil spells.

St John's wort was carried in amulets against witchcraft, thrown on hearths during storms, tied to cribs to avert changeling substitutions, and buried underneath cattle stall doorways and the thresholds of witches' houses. Until quite recently, women carried the plant during wartime, in the hope that it would prevent their violation. At the same time, soldiers smeared the ruddy sap on their rifle barrels to ensure unerring aim and accuracy.

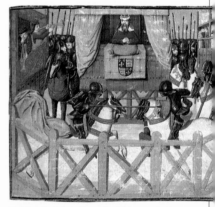

Knights jousting, from the 15th-century St Alban's Chronicle. *Medieval knights were allowed into tournaments only after swearing that they carried no St John's wort, as this would give them an unfair advantage.*

FROM PAGAN TO CHRISTIAN

The plant's scientific name, derived from the Greek *hypér*, "over", and *eíkon*, "picture image", indicates its association with pre-Christian religion and magic. Sprays of the plant were traditionally suspended over icons to drive away evil spirits. St John's wort was termed *piri* by the ancient Assyrians, who hung it on doorways during their ceremonies as a prophylactic against demons.

Coming into bloom on or around the summer solstice in a golden glow, the plant represented the summer and the solar rays dispersing all ill weather, darkness and evil. However, the early Christian missionaries in Europe found the plant consecrated to Balder, who represented, in their eyes, the spirits of darkness that fought against the sun. Rededicated to St John the Baptist, the plant was now held to have arisen from the drops of this saint's blood. As a result, St John's wort bled on the anniversary of the saint's beheading. When held up to the light, translucent oil glands give the leaves a perforated appearance. Satan himself, it was said, had wrathfully pierced these small holes, since the blood of St John in

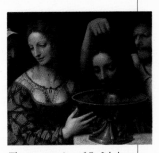

The presentation of St John's head to Herod, by Bernadino Luini (1480–1532).

the form of the pressed red juice had stood in the way of his imps. Consequently, St John's wort was hung in windows and doorways to avert thunderstorms, demons and the spirits of the dead.

---

effective in treating mild, symptomatic, reactive depressions, anxiety, nervous unrest, insomnia, neuralgia, psychotic disturbances, nervous headaches and migraine. Depressive disorders due to brain convulsions, nervous breakdown, arteriosclerosis of the cerebral blood vessels and climacteric conditions have all been successfully treated with St John's wort. Like most antidepressives, St John's wort becomes increasingly active only after several weeks of usage.

Taken internally, the plant tonifies circulation, stimulates the glands of the stomach, liver and gall, and is used to treat nervous stomachs, dyspepsia, diarrhoea, and catarrhal stomach ailments accompanied by gaseous heart burn. However, St John's wort is potentially dangerous in large amounts and should really only be used internally under expert supervision. St John's wort also makes the user abnormally sensitive to light.

An oil-based, balsamic ointment made from the leaves and flowers is rubbed on sprains, swellings, cramped muscles, lumbago, and other arthritic and rheumatic areas. In a fomentation (warm lotion) or ointment, the plant soothes and heals wounds, bruises, burns, insect bites, shingles, ulcers, fistula, sunburn and other skin irritations.

When combined with yarrow, St John's wort is used to treat bedwetting in children, mild mucosal infections of the head, chest and lung, kidney stones and bladder ailments. Combined with aloe, it is prescribed for liver congestion and mixed with mistletoe it stimulates monthly bleeding. St John's wort has also been used to treat epilepsy, blood effusion, anaemia, fever, sciatica, jaundice, gout and intestinal worms.

Walnut *Juglans regia*

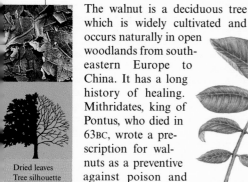

Dried leaves
Tree silhouette

The walnut is a deciduous tree which is widely cultivated and occurs naturally in open woodlands from south-eastern Europe to China. It has a long history of healing. Mithridates, king of Pontus, who died in 63BC, wrote a pre-scription for wal-nuts as a preventive against poison and infections, and the Greeks used walnuts to treat rabies and intestinal worms.

Walnut kernels have a deli-cious milky taste and are used in various confections and pas-tries; the young fruits are made into pickles and the ground shells added to spices. A decoction of the green husks has long been used as a dye for dark brown hair, while the decocted, crushed leaves yield an insect repellent. The oil and wood are used in the man-ufacture of food and soaps.

The walnut tree is rich in tannins which bind proteins in the skin and the mucus membranes, increasing the firmness and resiliency of the tissues. As a tea, gargle or wash, walnut leaves are prescribed for diar-rhoea, irritated gastroin-testinal systems and inflamma-tions of the gums, mouth and throat. Walnut teas are also used to allevi-ate symptoms of withdrawal when eliminating coffee from the diet.

As a compress, the decocted leaves are applied to inflamed eyelids and abscesses, frostbite, rashes, acne, eczema, fungal and other skin diseases. The leaves should be collected in June and quickly dried.

Because walnut is rich in vitamin C, walnut teas and baths were once exten-sively used for treating scurvy in chil-dren and also as a salve, rubbed on scrofulous sores. The root was used to make a strong purgative for treating headaches and fever, and the inner bark a mild laxative, without producing intestinal cramps and dependency.

Foot-baths are prescribed for exces-sive sweating of the feet and sitting-baths of walnut and oak bark are used for haemorrhoids and skin eruptions. As a home remedy, the plant was also used to treat rheumatism, diabetes, gout, colic, kidney pain, anaemia, jaun-dice, heavy menstrual bleeding, as a blood "cleanser" and to expel worms. However, individuals with sensitive stomachs may experience nausea and vomiting as a reaction to walnut and other tannic plants.

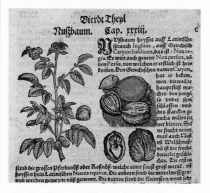

A walnut branch and kernel from the German Kreutzerbuch, *written by Lonitzer in 1557.*

Lovage *Levisticum officinale*

Lovage is native to southern Europe and Iran, and was a panacea in ancient Liguria. Praised by the botanist and medic Dioscorides, lovage was cultivated in Carolingian cloister gardens, and later became a popular garden plant. Often combined with anise and fennel, it was considered an important remedy for jaundice.

Diuretic, stimulant and carminative properties mean that lovage is commonly used in teas to treat digestive problems. Lovage teas are also used for coughs and hoarseness, to loosen mucus-congested respiratory tracts, kidneys, liver and spleen, to lighten heavy breathing and alleviate bronchitis. Migraine, hysteria, edema, heart ailments and rheumatoid arthritis have all been tackled with lovage.

Fresh, macerated lovage, at times mixed with ground ivy, is applied in a linen to raw throats and swollen thyroid glands. Lovage has antiseptic and antibiotic properties and is used in poultices for pustulent wounds and swellings. As an antidote to poison, lovage is recommended for the overuse of nicotine and alcohol.

Dried root

The ancient Egyptians added lovage to sauces for grilled fish and it is primarily used today as a spice and flavouring for meat, sauces and stews. The seeds or leafy stems are also added to biscuits, soups, salads, liqueurs and potpourris. Lovage makes a soothing bath additive, a deodorizing skin wash and decoction to remove freckles.

Overuse may cause inflammation of the kidney and urinary tract, and reduced kidney activity. Lovage also induces menstruation and lactation in nursing mothers, and should not be taken by pregnant women.

CONSECRATED HERBS

In Austria lovage has long been carried in processions on Corpus Christi to be blessed, and then used as a prophylactic to ward off stormy weather and evil spirits. On St John's Day, it used to be served in milk to cattle and three crosses of the plant were set up in the corners of fields as protection against malevolent witches.

Serbian, Slovak and Ruthenian maidens carried the consecrated root for success in love, and Slovenian brides used the herb to divine whether their marriage was to be peaceful. As a cure for unrequited love, the root was buried when the sun stood in the zodiacal sign of Aries, and was then dug up and worn as an amulet.

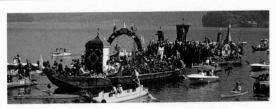
A waterborne Corpus Christi procession, in which the boats are decorated with lovage as well as other flowers and herbs.

High mallow *Malva sylvestris/Malva neglecta*

The flowers and leaves of the high mallow, collected in June and July, should be used fresh rather than dried. High mallow tea is recommended for coughs due to colds, extreme hoarseness and mild diarrhoea. As a soothing wash and gargle, an infusion of the herb serves as a palliative for inflammations of the gums, mouth and throat.

The whole plant, especially the root, abounds in mucilage, and has been used as an expectorant, demulcent and febrifuge in treating internal inflammations, irritations of the air passage, upper respiratory tract infections with heavy mucous secretion, bronchitis and tonsillitis. For a tea or gargle, 2 teaspoonfuls of the plant are left to steep in a cup of lukewarm water for some 5–10 hours while occasionally being stirred, and then strained. High mallow, mixed with equal parts of primrose root, provides an excellent expectorant and anti-inflammatory tea that can be used for coughs in children.

The herb and root, cooked with fennel and anise seeds and taken with wine, soothe intestinal and bladder pain, and soften hard stools. As a folk remedy the leaves, prepared with barley as a soup, have been used to strengthen weak intestines and to heal intestinal ulcers. The herb, boiled in milk, was also taken for consumption and stomach ulcers. The freshly macerated leaves, roots and seeds were applied in a compress to render swollen glands and other swellings soft and flexible.

Asthma, coughs, whooping cough and inflammations of the throat were treated with the hot vapours given off by an infusion of high mallow, elder, chamomile flowers, senna leaves and some ammoniacal salts as a preservative. Vapour baths using high mallow flowers have also been used in treating ear ailments.

The leaves of high mallow were eaten as a vegetable by the Egyptians, Romans, Chinese and Greeks, but were forbidden to the Pythagoreans, who considered them to be sacred. The Anglo-Saxons also cultivated the plant as a vegetable and the fruits, termed "cheeses", were avidly eaten by children. These fruits are the origin of the plant's other common name, the "cheese flower". High mallow flowers were also planted around Anglo-Saxon graves and the fibre was woven into a fabric. The Hungarians used the roots to induce abortion. They also buried high mallow leaves under stable doors to prevent witches from stealing milk. In medieval Silesia, high mallow was used to divine whether a woman was to have children. The urine of the woman was poured on the plant and if it withered within three days the woman was infertile.

Horehound *Marrubium vulgare*

The whole plant is medicinal and should be gathered before flowering in June. Horehound promotes perspiration and the flow of urine. Taken as a hot tea or syrup, it is a well-known remedy for sore throats, coughs, chronic pulmonary catarrh, bronchitis and stomach catarrh. As a cold infusion, horehound makes an excellent tonic for general debility.

An alternative remedy for chronic catarrh, bronchitis and coughs is a shot glass of the fresh plant cooked in wine and taken three times a day. The dried herb, warmed in wine and honey, is a remedy for weak intestinal tissue.

Washing with horehound decoctions removes dandruff in children. As a folk remedy, horehound has provided relief for asthma, jaundice, nervous heart rhythm, inflammations of the liver, tuberculosis and skin diseases. An ointment from the leaves was used to soothe itching and cleanse wounds. The fresh herb, boiled in water, was applied in a linen compress to treat muffled hearing. The plant was also used to regulate menstruation and to ease the painful aftereffects of infant delivery.

Dried herb

Milk thistle *Silybum marianum*

Infusions of the fruits of milk thistle (also known as holy thistle) have been used as a household remedy for mild digestive and chest ailments, edema, jaundice, leucorrhoea, and as a blood purifier. The fruits are effective in treating sciatica, spitting of blood; and coughing and blood vomiting in cases where these are symptoms of liver and spleen ailments. They also stimulate the gall and soothe the pain of gallstone-colic.

The plant contains silymarin, which protects the liver from infections such as viral hepatitis and helps to regenerate damaged livers and stimulate the production of liver cells.

The mashed fruits are also effective in preventing liver damage from the ingestion of solvents and other toxins. As a long-term remedy, teas of the plant are beneficial for those with cirrhosis.

Silymarin is poorly absorbed by the digestive system, so the drug is most effective taken through the skin. The concentrated doses necessary in a tea, however, produce no adverse reactions. As a treatment for ulcers of the limbs and varicose veins, the pulverized fruits are applied in a compress.

Fruits

Lemon balm *Melissa officinalis*

Dried herb

Also known as garden balm, sweet balm or cure-all (it has been used as a household remedy for problems ranging from flatulence to anaemia), lemon balm is collected before flowering, between early June and late summer. The citrus-like odour is nearly lost upon drying. Lemon balm has a calming effect on the nervous system, and is recommended in cases of unrest brought about by insomnia and for other nervous ailments. These calming properties have also been found useful in treating toothaches and earaches, cramp-like heart and gastrointestinal ailments, vomiting (especially during pregnancy), extreme fatigue and unsettling dreams. Lemon balm has even been used to treat the illusion of illness, having been recommended by 9th-century Arab physicians in cases of hypochondria. They also prescribed it for depression.

Lemon balm contains vitamins C and E, and beta-carotene, which have known anticarcinogenic properties. Vitamin E also helps ameliorate cardiac damage.

The essential oil is a powerful germicide, which makes it an excellent anti-putrescent dressing for wounds. The oil's hydrocarbons contain little free oxygen, which asphyxiates aerobic bacteria, and the resins dry upon contact, neatly sealing the wound. A cream containing the plant's extract has been marketed for treating cold sores, lesions and related conditions caused by the herpes simplex virus.

Used as a body rub, the spirits have a tonic effect and shore up the body's defences against seasonal colds and other infections. Washing with lemon balm tea or infusion conditions the skin, and the fresh plants, crushed or in lotion, cool and ease the pain of rheumatism, gout, neuralgia, migraine, bruises, insect bites and paralyzed muscles.

SCENT AND FLAVOUR

Lemon balm has been a popular plant among Mediterranean beekeepers for more than 2,000 years. The odour of the essential oil is similar to that of a pheromone (scent-hormone) produced by bees. Hives are rubbed with the plant to keep the bees within close range, especially during swarming. Rural beekeepers also plant balm to attract the bees, and smear their hands with the juice

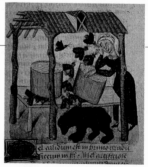

Beekeepers collecting honey, from the 15th-century French herbal, Dioscorides Tractatus de Herbis.

before retrieving the queen bee from the swarm.

The aroma of lemon balm is widely used and appreciated. A handful of fresh lemon balm leaves tied in a muslin bag and immersed in a bath imparts a refreshing, lemony scent to the water. The leaves are also added to potpourris and herb cushions and the oil to perfumes and liqueurs. A few leaves added to fruit juices, wine and iced tea add a cool, fragrant flavour.

Basil *Ocimum basilieum*

Basil is often referred to as sweet or garden basil, or more rarely, and archaically, as St Josephwort. It has mildly sedative, antiseptic, expectorant, anti-flatulent and laxative properties. For medicinal purposes only the freshly procured plant, gathered before flowering, should be used. When dried the pungent leaves have a peppery taste.

When taken as a tea, basil alleviates stomach spasms and cramps, chronic gastritis, indigestion and constipation. Basil tea has also been used as a blood purifier and to stimulate lactation in nursing mothers. As a gargle, the tea is used to treat thrush and inflammations of the throat.

A tincture of the camphoraceous oil is applied by brush or in a compress to injuries and badly healing wounds or suppurations. It may also be rubbed on

Dried herb

the temples to relieve headaches. The freshly crushed leaves, taken as a snuff or in a facial steam bath, are used for headaches and colds.

The fresh herb or seeds are cooked in white wine with a little honey as a digestive tonic and to reduce fevers. Fresh, minced basil leaves add a sweet, delicate pungency to tomato dishes, green salads, soft cheeses, vegetable soups and pesto sauce. The flavour of basil is increased when cooked, and as a digestive aid basil lends itself to thick, brown meat soups, sausage mixtures and other fatty dishes. It is extensively used in curries. Basil adds warmth to potpourris and aromatic sachets, and the essential oil is used in the preparation of commercial condiments, catsups, mustards, vinegars, cosmetics and perfumes.

FUNERARY HERBS

Sweet basil is indigenous to India and Iran. In India the plant is sacred to Vishnu and embodies his illustrious wife, Lakshmi. To destroy the plant fills the god with anguish and he therefore spurns the prayers of those who ravage the plant. Votaries of Vishnu use rosaries made of basil seeds and wear beads made of the root around the arms and neck. Basil is frequently grown near Hindu temples and homes, where it is used as a disinfectant and air-freshener. A basil leaf is

placed on the breast of the deceased before burial, which is then shown at heaven's gate to gain admittance.

In Iran and Malaysia basil is planted on graves, and in Egypt women scatter the flowers over graves. In ancient Greece basil was also a sign of grief and mourning, but in addition symbolized hate, poverty and misfortune. Although a staple in Greek kitchens, basil would not grow and thrive unless it was sown with cursing and abuse.

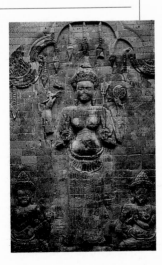

A 12th-century brick bas-relief of Lakshmi, from Angkor in Cambodia.

Plantain *Plantage lanceolata*

The plantain is also widely known as cuckoo's bread, waybread, ribwort, soldier's herb and ripple grass. A single plant produces some 14,000 seeds annually, which may account for its prolific and often pesty presence in lawns and pavement cracks. Designated as the "ruler of the road" because of its ubiquity, the plantain was believed to have great healing power by Alexander the Great and the ancient Greek medic and historian, Dioscorides. Plantain was one of nine sacred herbs of the Anglo-Saxons, who used it as a panacea for fevers, kidney diseases, poisonous bites, haemorrhoids, ulcers, wounds and many other ailments. Throughout Europe this apparently paltry weed was highly esteemed as a cure for everything from dysentery to the epidemics that accompanied famine and war. For country people, the crushed leaves or juice were a handy, effective remedy for burns, wounds, swellings and insect stings.

The fresh leaves are collected shortly before flowering and dried well. They are rich in mucilage and astringent tannins, have a styptic, anti-inflammatory effect, deter blood poisoning and hasten the healing of wounds, burns and scalded skin. The leaves, taken in a tea or cooked with sugar to a syrupy consistency, stimulate the appetite and have been used to alleviate gastritis, chronic diarrhoea, asthma, whooping cough, haemorrhoids, fever, consumption and epilepsy.

Plantain contains mucilage, salicylic acid, a tonifying bitter, potassium and other chemicals with antibiotic, anti-inflammatory, expectorant, capillary-resistant, soothing, mildly laxative, diuretic and astringent activities. Taken as either a tea or in syrup form, plantain is presently prescribed for inflammation of the throat and upper respiratory tract because of catarrh, bronchitis and other chronic pulmonary diseases. Plantain is especially recommended as a cough and flu medicine for children.

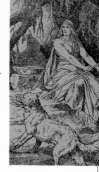

Plantain once embodied a spirit who ruled the way to the domain of Hel, the pre-Christian goddess of death, shown here in a 19th-century engraving.

As a folk remedy, plantain teas have also been used to ease nose bleeding, bloody urine and vomiting, hypermenorrhoea, weak and ulcerous bladder and liver conditions, and to expel mawworms. Plantain is a staple in seasonal blood-purifying and anti-mucoid tea formulas.

The soaked seeds or fresh juice can be thinned with chamomile tea and applied in a compress to ulcers, headaches and eye and ear inflammations. After being boiled for 5 minutes in milk, the plant extract is used as a cosmetic on sore and rough skin.

Oak *Quercus robur* and *Quercus petraea*

Although the leaves, acorns and galls of oak are all medicinal, it is only the shiny bark of young branches that is primarily collected today. The young bark, free of algae and lichen, is easily removed in the spring and quickly dried. An infusion of the bark is recommended as a gargle for infections of the mouth, throat and gums. Infusions of the bark have also been used to treat inflammations of the mucous lining of the gastrointestinal system, acute diarrhoea, dysentery, bedwetting, bleeding of the urinary and gastrointestinal tracts and hypermenorrhoea.

A handful of the bark boiled in 2 pints (1 litre) of milk is an excellent antidote for the ingestion of poisonous berries, mushrooms and strychnine. However, strong oak tea disturbs the stomach and the plant should not be taken by those with nervous intestinal conditions, inflamed kidneys or distended livers.

The whole plant is rich in catechin tannins which have astringent, antiseptic, styptic, and anti-inflammatory properties. Oak is also active against zymogenic bacteria and has been used as a quinine substitute for alleviating malarial fever. The acorns, powdered and roasted, yield a coffee substitute which has been used as a household remedy for weak digestive organs, anaemia, nervous conditions and tuberculosis. The powdered bark may be taken as a snuff to stop nosebleeds.

Used as a wash, repeated infusions of the leaves or bark temper heavy sweating of the feet, bed sores, skin irritations and minor haemorrhages. Warm baths with a bark decoction relieve haemorrhoids, ulcers, chronic eczema, chilblains and vaginal problems.

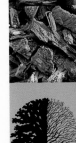

Gall
Dried bark
Tree silhouette

SACRED OAKS

As the largest tree in Europe, the oak symbolizes endurance, fertility and eternal life. Giant old oak trees were believed to be coexistent with the creation of the world and offered protection from lightning. The Israelites and all European peoples once carried out their religious rites under great oaks and in oak groves. Christian missionaries waged a fierce battle against these sacred trees, which were often associated with pagan deities of thunder, sky and rain.

Yet the oak retained its importance long after Europe was converted to Christianity. St Columba and other Irish saints appropriated the tree as their own. Medieval oak trees served as territorial boundary markers and English kings planted an oak tree at their coronations.

The oak leaf and flower were carved with exquisite beauty and fidelity in medieval churches. Oak was used to carve religious images and acorns were placed in the hands of those about to be buried. Coffins were made of oak and pall-bearers carried oaken staffs.

People held solemn processions to holy oaks each year. The fairy world was believed to dwell in the roots of oak trees, and Joan of Arc was thought to have received her sword and banner from the fairy spirit of an oak.

Rosemary *Rosmarinus officinalis*

Dried herb

Rosemary stimulates and strengthens the circulatory and nervous systems and is widely approved for treating flatulence, satiety, minor gastrointestinal cramps and low blood pressure. It contains chemicals which have astringent, anti-flatulent and sweat-inducing properties. The essential oil is antagonistic to the presence of calcium, which makes it a smooth-muscle relaxant, as well as having antioxidant, antiseptic and antimicrobial properties.

Oil of rosemary is used in salves, liniments and embrocations as a stimulant to treat gout, muscular rheumatism, nervous headaches, neuralgia, muscular aches, sprains, tired limbs and swollen feet. When added to baths, rosemary extracts help to stimulate and tone the skin, while oil of rosemary can be used as a hair conditioner, which leaves the hair lustrous and manageable, controls dandruff and is said to prevent hair-loss.

Rosemary can be taken in wine or alcohol to treat edema, inflamed and torpid livers, nervous conditions and as a heart stimulant. Arab physicians used rosemary to restore speech after a stroke and in China it is prescribed for headaches, insomnia and mental fatigue. Hungarian Water, the main ingredient of which is rosemary, was extensively used to treat apoplexy, paralyzed limbs and other nervous disorders. Rosemary tea is a traditional autumn and winter tonic for the convalescent.

As a household remedy, it has been used to treat anaemia, congestions due to colds, halitosis, childhood tantrums, dizziness and epilepsy.

Having been brought over the Alps into northern Europe by the first Christian monks, rosemary was popular in monastic gardens for its medicinal properties, and was strewn in chests of clothing to ward off moths or burnt in sickrooms as an aromatic disinfectant. It was used to decorate halls during the Yuletide feast. Rosemary aids weak digestion and, with thyme, its fresh subtle flavour is a natural supplement to roast meats. It also imparts a pungent flavour to biscuits, jams, fruit salads, soft cheeses, mushrooms and vegetable soups. The dried culinary herb, soaked for several hours, should be used sparingly. The essential oil is used in the manufacture of eau de cologne, perfumes and vermouth, and bees that are nurtured on rosemary provide an excellent aromatic honey.

Throughout the Roman Empire, rosemary was used to adorn the pillar-images of the protective household spirits (or Lares, shown here on a shrine from the atrium of the House of the Vetii in Pompeii).

THE SYMBOL OF REMEMBRANCE

In ancient Athens and Rome rosemary sprigs, as a symbol of the soul's immortality, were placed in the hands of the deceased and burned as incense at funerals and other religious rites. During the Shepherds' festival held in April to commemorate the founding of Rome, rosemary was burned to purify sacred groves, flocks and fountains. The herb had more than just a metaphorical link with remembrance and commemoration, however: Greek students twined rosemary sprigs in their hair before taking exams in order to stimulate their memory and mental prowess.

Because of its reputation for strengthening the memory, rosemary also became the emblem for fidelity between lovers. As a result, in both Greece and Rome rosemary was used in marriage ceremonies as well as funerals, and guests of honour at feasts were crowned with rosemary garlands. In post-classical Europe, too, a notable feature of rosemary has been its use at both marriages and funerals. As a symbol of eternal devotion, rosemary sprigs are still worn by the bridegroom in his lapel and as a bridal wreath or bouquet by the bride. The bridesmaids, marriage guests and post-nuptial food table are also frequently adorned with rosemary.

Sir Thomas More wrote: "As for Rosmarine, I lett it run all over my garden walls, not onlie because my bees love it, but because it is the herb sacred to remembrance, and, therefore, to friendship; whence a sprig of it hath a dumb language that maketh it to be the chosen emblem of our funeral wakes and in our buriall grounds." Rosemary bouquets are still often borne in funeral processions, placed in the hands of the dead, cast on the coffin and planted on graves. In Britain the herb is used each 11 November to commemorate those who died in the two world wars.

Rosemary has also been used to decorate baptismal fonts, and was worn by godfathers at sacramental rites. In early Christian legends rosemary represented the Virgin Mary, because it sheltered her during her flight into Egypt.

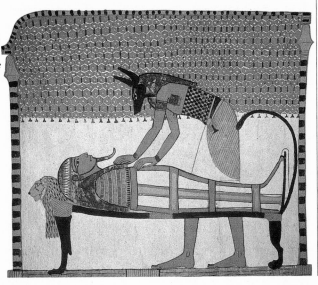

The association of rosemary with funerary rites dates back at least as far as the ancient Egyptians, who used the herb to embalm the bodies of the dead. Anubis, the Egyptian god of the dead and patron deity of embalmers, is shown here on a wall of the Tomb of Sennedjem in the process of embalming a mummy. The tomb lies in the Valley of the Kings, and dates from the 19th Dynasty of the New Kingdom, c.1320–1200BC.

Sweet brier *Rosa canina*

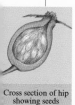

Cross section of hip showing seeds

The ripe, red fruits or hips of sweet brier (also known as dog rose and wild rose) are gathered in late autumn after the first frost, rapidly dried and kept in tightly closed containers. Rose hips have a high content of vitamin C and also contain vitamins A, B and E, as well as iron and phosphorus. Vitamin C helps form connective tissue, such as collagen, and is vital for the healing of wounds, the working of allergic responses and the production of adrenal hormones. Vitamin C is also essential to strengthen the immune system against infections. Consequently, rose-hip tea provides an excellent preventive medicine during the flu season, and is recommended for fevers, colds and related infections, general debility and badly healing wounds.

As a medicine, rose hip is usually combined with other plant drugs, lime or linden flowers being an excellent choice. Rose hips may be prepared by removing the achenes – or "seeds" – and hairs from the urn-shaped receptacle or hip (although the achenes themselves are of medicinal value and add a vanilla flavour to the tea). Rose hips have tonic, mildly astringent and anti-flatulent properties. The tea also has a diuretic effect, without irritating the kidneys. As an infusion or syrup, rose hip has been used as a spring remedy and, prepared with sugar or milk, to treat diarrhoea, scurvy, stomach cramps, and kidney or bladder stones. The soaked achenes or pips have been taken for edema, gout, rheumatism and sciatica. The entire hips, taken raw, act as a deworming agent.

Rose hip marmalade stimulates the appetite and, as a purée, rose hips are used for desserts and sauces. The delicately flavoured petals are added to conserves, cakes and sweets and, distilled, are extensively used in Middle Eastern cookery and perfumes.

FIRE AND SLUMBER

In pre-Christian Europe the wood of the brier was used for pyres to cremate the dead. Because of its scarlet fruit, the plant was consecrated to Loki, the Norse fire god, and later became associated with the Christian devil.

The Norse god Odin pricked Brunhilde with a magic rose thorn or, in another version, laid rose galls under her head, plunging her into profound sleep before surrounding her with a wall of flame. Rose galls are formed on the brier by wasps. Termed the "nest of Mother Helle" and "sleep apples", they were put under pillows to induce prophetic dreams and placed in cribs to protect infants from bewitchment and cramps.

The sleep of Brunhilde, from Die Walkure, *painted by Arthur Rackham in 1910.*

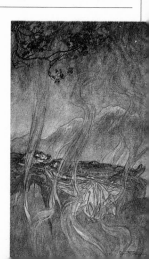

Sage *Salvia officinalis*

The medicinal properties of sage were discovered, according to Greek legend, by the hero Cadmus, to whom the leaves were offered each year in a religious ceremony. In medieval Europe, sage was employed in brewing ale, making love, magic and as a tisane for prolonging life. With the aid of sage and some words of power, young women were able to see their future husbands.

Sage was once an important medicinal herb but is at present primarily used as a gargle for inflamed gums, bad breath, minor sore throats, laryngitis, tonsillitis and other inflammations and infections of the mouth and throat. The leaves are rubbed on to the teeth as a mouth deodorant and gum strengthener, and smoked to alleviate wheezing or short breath. They can also be used as a wash to dispel head lice and to cure mange. Sage provides an aromatic rinse for darkening grey hair, while the essential oil is used in the manufacture of perfumes, soaps, face powders and condiments.

Dried leaves

Once considered the food of the gods, sage is popular in stuffings and sauces for lamb, fatty meats, poultry and fish, as well as soups, cheese, curds and vegetable dishes. Sage should not be taken by pregnant women, and prolonged and excessive internal use may result in adverse reactions.

Sage tea is a traditional spring tonic for strengthening weak constitutions and cleansing the liver and kidney. It has been used as a household remedy for coughs and colds, influenza, rheumatism and to inhibit lactation during weaning. The medicinal effect of sage depends very much on the dosage: a weak decoction of the tea increases perspiration, whereas a strong decoction arrests perspiration.

As a compress or salve, sage has been used in treating gout, stroke, suppurating wounds, paralytic and trembling limbs, and lingering ulcers of the limbs and feet. When added to a bath, a strong decoction of the leaves stimulates and cleanses the skin and scalp, and soothes tired muscles. In facial steam baths, sage has an astringent effect on the skin and is a traditional remedy for severe head colds.

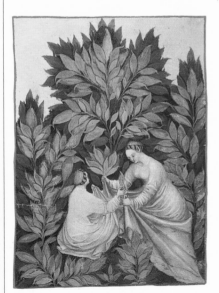

Sage should always be gathered in fine weather, as in this 15th-century French illustration.

Elder *Sambucus nigra*

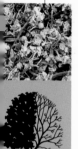

Dried flowers
Tree silhouette

The elder has an impressive range of alternative names, including the boon-tree, dogtree, Judas tree, God's stinking tree, pipe tree and popgun tree. Several of the elder's names refer to the hollow stems of the plant, among them the common name, which is thought to derive from the Anglo-Saxon *aeld*, meaning kindle, because hollow lengths of wood are especially good for starting fires.

Although the whole of the plant has been employed medicinally, the flowers are the main parts used today. The blossoms should be carefully gathered in dry weather when the plant is in early bloom, between May and June, and quickly dried.

Elder exhibits analgesic, antibacterial, anti-inflammatory, hypotensive and spasmolytic activity. The ripe fruits are rich in minerals and vitamins A, B, C and J (which relieves pulmonary inflammation). Elder tea has been used as a diuretic, a mild stimulant, an emetic (to induce vomiting) and a cathartic. Taken hot and in copious amounts, the tea induces perspiration, which is helpful in treating feverish colds. Its mildly diuretic properties come to the fore when it is less strongly brewed and taken in lukewarm sips, when it also stimulates the body's defence against

colds and flus. Elder forms the basis for many different tea remedies taken for chills and cold-like diseases, in which it is combined with chamomile, lime or linden flowers and other ingredients. Taken on a long-term, regular basis, elder teas relieve rheumatic pain and lengthen the intervals between rheumatic attacks. They have been popular household remedies for childhood asthma, edema, bronchitis, sinusitis, erysipelas, cystitis and inflamed urinary mucus membranes. They have also been used as a mild laxative and to promote menses.

Elder infusions can be taken both internally and externally to treat gout and to clear congestions of the liver, kidney and spleen. As a compress, the blossoms are used to soothe the pain of boils and ulcers and the macerated flowers are boiled in milk with saffron and applied in a plaster or poultice to ease the pain of rheumatic limbs and inflamed joints.

Prepared as a juice or purée, the berries are taken to treat neuralgia, sciatica, constipation and diarrhoea, as a demulcent to soothe coughs and congested colds, and to stimulate digestive and circulatory activity. However, the unripened berries are slightly toxic and their juice, when uncooked, induces nausea, diarrhoea and vomiting. The

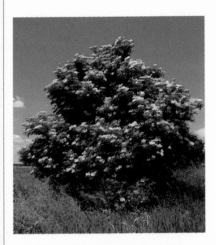

The wood of the mature elder is valued by craftsman, and its Latin name may derive from the Greek sambuke, *a wooden-framed harp. However, elder was not used to make cradles, in case the spirit of the tree hurt the child.*

juice can be used externally, prepared in lard or cream, as an effective ointment for burns and scalds. The leaves can also be prepared in an ointment for burns, scalds, bruises, sprains and wounds, and in a cold-infusion wash to soothe irritated skin.

The fresh, honey-scented flowers provide a refreshing summer beverage with a pleasant, distinctive flavour. The berries or flowers are added to jams, jellies, milk dishes, chutneys, fritters, wine and ordinary, non-healing teas. The flowers are used in facial steam baths or mixed with yogurt or cucumber juice to cleanse and soften dry or oily skin. Elder flower water provides a mild astringent skin lotion and is added to almond-oil based complexion creams. A tisane of the flowers is a pleasant, astringent after-shave lotion.

TREE OF THE EARTH

In Baltic–Slavic countries the elder tree was the dwelling place of Puschkayt, a deity of the earth for whom food offerings were placed at the base of the elder in the evening. In northern Europe the plant was the dwelling place of an elder-mother called Holda, who was a death and fertility goddess. Bearing elder saplings, women danced in her honour during the Candlemas feast in February and struck any man nearing the dance ground. Destroying an elder tree caused agony to this goddess, and to prevent her from avenging injuries to the plant, her permission was always requested before removing any branches.

Collected at midnight on St John's Eve, the plant was a prophylactic against storms, thieves, evil spirits and magic. Preparing elder-flower fritters, which were a treat on St John's Day, pleased the elder-mother and prevented discord between married couples. Anointing the eyes with the inner bark or floating the burning pith in a glass of water on Christmas Eve revealed any witches and sorcerers nearby.

In Germany, coffins used to be made of elder and elder-wood crosses and wreaths were placed in the grave. In northern England and the Tyrol, elder bushes,

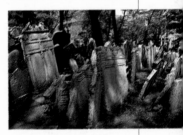

The old Jewish cemetery in Prague is filled with elders, a legacy of the historical link between this tree and death.

trimmed in the form of a cross, were planted upon fresh graves. The elder has variously been claimed as the wood of the cross on which Christ was crucified, and as the tree from which Judas hanged himself.

Dandelion *Taraxacum officinale*

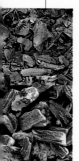

Dried stem
and leaves
Dried root

The leaves, flowers and roots are gathered before flowering (April–May), although the autumn roots have a higher content of inulin, beneficial in treating diabetes and anaemia due to liver malfunctions. Dandelion contains taraxacin and choline, which stimulate liver cell metabolism, and a sugar, laevulose, which is easily assimilated by diabetics. The plant is also rich in vitamins A, B-complex, C and E, as well as calcium, iron and potassium. Individuals prone to or suffering from liver and gall ailments, rheumatism, anaemia and diabetes benefit from a 4–6 week seasonal treatment using dandelion.

Infusions of the plant stimulate the flow of bile and promote digestion.

As such, they are a gentle remedy for flatulence, atonic syspepsia and disturbances in gall bladder secretion. Dandelion tinctures and deliciously bitter teas have been used as household remedies to treat eczema and skin eruptions, edema, gout and varicose veins.

The plant can be applied in plasters to swollen glands and skin diseases, and the milky juice of the stem is rubbed on to warts. The juice of the root is highly active and may be combined, as a spring and autumn remedy, with nettle and watercress juices. The roots are prepared like asparagus and taken as a spring remedy to improve liver, gall and pancreatic functioning. The juice of the roots is a cosmetic lotion. The tender, macerated leaves can also safely be used in a face pack on skin impurities, although, as a dye, dandelion leaves turn fabric deep magenta.

A UNIVERSAL METER

Because the flowers open at five o'clock in the morning and close in the evening, the dandelion is sometimes called the shepherd's clock; one of 150 names given to the plant by the Swiss. The downy puff balls serve as a barometer: the seeds flying off when there is no wind is a sign of impending rain.

The feathery seed balls are consulted as oracles. When the fruits are blown away, the remaining seeds determine one's lifespan or number of offspring. Blowing on the puff ball three times with the result that one feather remains indicates that the user's sweetheart is thinking of him or her. Then the enamoured can pick one of the blossoms and send a message by whispering to the flower and blowing toward the loved one. Children use dandelion stems in games, as musical instruments and as necklaces and bracelets.

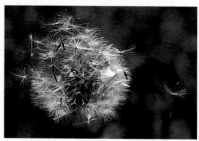

A dandelion spreading its seeds on the wind.

Lime or linden *Tilia cordata* and *Tilia platyphyllos*

The flowers and parchment-like bracts of the lime or linden tree are at their peak, and should be collected, as soon as they blossom. They are dried at a low temperature and kept in tightly-closed containers. The spring sap can also be used: it purifies the blood, dispels kidney stones and is a face and hair lotion.

Lime tea promotes perspiration, alleviates coughs, hoarseness, sore throats, chills and congestion due to colds and flu, and also stimulates the body's defence system so that feverish colds, especially in children, are swiftly surmounted. Regular and strong infusions of lime tea are an excellent prophylactic at the onset of cold symptoms, either on their own or with yarrow flowers and sage. When mixed with chamomile and elder flowers, lime combats flu and, if taken regularly with coltsfoot leaves, it provides an effective remedy for bronchitis.

Lime has antispasmodic and mildly tranquillizing and sedative properties. It can be used in teas and baths in order to relieve rheumatic pain, nervous tension, anxiety and insomnia. It also helps calm excitable, hyperactive children. In European folk medicine, the decoction of the bark has been used as an emollient and demulcent dressing for burns and wounds, and to alleviate stomach cramps, halitosis, and urinary pains.

Tree silhouette

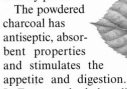

The powdered charcoal has antiseptic, absorbent properties and stimulates the appetite and digestion. In European herbal medicine, the charcoal has long been used to treat colic, diarrhoea, flatulency, heartburn, stomach catarrh, night sweats and fever. Sprinkled on pustulent wounds, the powdered charcoal absorbs toxins so that injuries are able to heal properly.

As a wash or facial steam bath, infusions of the flowers improve circulation to the skin. The flowers are the source of an excellent honey and may be distilled to make an aftershave lotion. In teas the honey-scented flowers provide a soothing, relaxing after-dinner and nocturnal beverage, but prolonged, excessive use can damage the heart.

LOVE AND DEATH

The lime or linden tree is a symbol of exalted, divine power, valour and victory. The ancient Greeks and the Slavs regarded it as the habitation of their goddess of love, and in Germany it was the haunt of dwarfs, fairies and dragons. The tree was extensively planted in courtyards, markets, cemeteries and pilgrimage chapels devoted to the Virgin Mary. Judgements would be passed under sacred, old lindens. In the Somme, before World War I, a bridal couple would walk under two lime trees that had grown together in order to secure a blissful marriage.

The lime is also a tree of ill fortune. In old Norse and Germanic myth, Sigurd or Siegfried bathes in the blood of a dragon he has slain to make himself invincible, but a lime leaf falls on his shoulder, making him vulnerable to Hagen's spear. Nevertheless, Sigurd is buried beneath a lime, since it was regarded as the tree of resurrection.

Nettle *Urtica dioica* and *Urtica urens*

Dried herb

The nettle is rich in vitamins A and C, carotene, acetylcholine, histamine, magnesium, phosphorous, potassium, calcium and other minerals. The high vitamin, mineral and plant-hormone content increases body metabolism. Nettle also has astringent, tonic and strong diuretic properties, presently utilized in treating urinary disorders caused by enlarged prostates and reduced heart and kidney activity. The leaves and tops are collected in late spring and early summer. The roots are at their best in June and July. The plants must be collected with scissors and gloves, but boiling in water removes their sting.

Nettle stimulates the gastrointestines, pancreas and gall. Its multiple active constituents make it beneficial for a range of diseases. Nettle teas have been home remedies for arthritis, gout, shortness of breath, phlegm-congested lungs, bronchitis, nervous eczema and haemorrhoids.

The pulverized root, cooked with sugar in sweet violet syrup, is an excellent remedy for whooping cough and inflamed throats. Decoctions of the plant help lower blood sugar levels and blood pressure, and increase the number of red blood cells. Rich in copper, iron and silicylic acid, which improve the condition of the blood, nettle is used to treat secondary anaemia, chlorosis, diabetes, uterine haemorrhages, hives, and to diminish menstrual and other bleeding.

The bruised leaves are applied as a poultice to alleviate burns, scabs, wounds, indurate spleens and neuralgia. The leaves may be used as a gargle to soothe toothache and in foot-baths for rheumatism, or they can be burned and inhaled to treat asthma. People have been beaten with fresh nettles as a treatment for rheumatism, paralysis, pleurisy, measles and scarlet fever.

The juice, applied with a stiff brush or massaged into the scalp, removes dandruff and invigorates the hair. Applied with face packs or pads, nettle infusions promote a clear complexion.

PAIN AND PROTECTION

The Indians believe that the nettle is a symbol of Vasuki, a giant serpent which let its venom fall on the plant, giving it the ability to cause a burning pain. Nevertheless, nettle is a popular

A carving of Vasuki from Amritsar, India.

medicine in India, and decoctions of the plant are administered for kidney disorders, fevers and chills, and to arrest haemorrhaging and excessive menstruation.

In Peru nettle was used as a whip to punish adulterous women, and in old Ireland nettle-wielding boys ran wildly about once a year striking anyone they could reach with impunity. In Hungary, cows were hit on Whitsuntide Eve with nettle, as a prophylactic against pernicious witches.

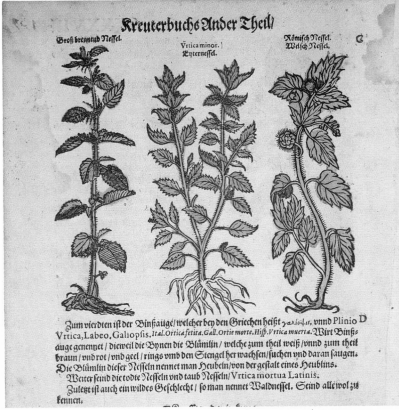

Kreuterbuchs Ander Theil/

Groß brennend Nessel.   Vrtica minor. | Römisch Nessel.
              Eyternessel.   Welsch Nessel,

Zum vierdten ist der Binßauge/welcher bey den Griechen heißt γαλιοψιs, vnnd Plinio D
Vrtica, Labeo, Galiopsis. Ital. Ortica fetita. Gall. Ortie morte, Hiß. Vrtica muerta. Wirt Binß=
auge genennet / dieweil die Bynen die Blümlin / welche zum theil weiß /vnnd zum theil
braun / vnd rot / vnd geel / rings vmb den Stengel her wachsen/suchen vnd daran saugen.
Die Blümlin dieser Nesseln nennet man Heubeln/von der gestalt eines Heublins.
Weiter seind die todte Nesseln vnd taub Nesseln/Vrtica mortua Latinis.
Zuletzt ist auch ein wildes Geschlecht / so man nennet Waldnessel. Seind alle wol zu
kennen.

Three nettles from the 15th-century
Kreutzerbuch, *by Lonitzer. In pre-industrial*
Europe, a beer, taken for rheumatism, was
brewed from nettles. The plant was cultivated as
a garden crop, used as a green dye and provided
fibre for cloth, sheets and fishing nets.

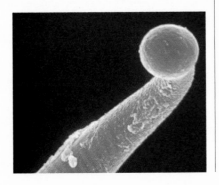

The hairs on the leaves of the stinging nettle
have globular, silicified (fragile and quartzlike)
tips which break off when brushed. The resulting
sharp point injects histamine, which causes
allergic reactions, and acetylcholine, a neuro-
transmitter ordinarily found in nerves, which
amplifies the sensation of pain.

Mullein *Verbascum densiflorum*

Dried herb

Also known as flannel leaf and velvet dock, mullein is an old favourite of poachers, who used to scatter its toxic seeds on water at night in order to stupefy fish.

The leaves, roots and flowers all contain saponins, flavonoid glycosides, mucilage and other constituents which produce a number of beneficial effects. Between them they have antibiotic, anti-inflammatory, antispasmodic, expectorant, astringent, calmative and mildly diuretic properties.

Mullein is especially effective in treating colds, coughs and phlegm-congestion in upper respiratory tracts. As a catarrh remedy, it is prepared in tea mixtures with plantain, oregano and sage leaves; with hollyhock and chamomile flowers; and with the pulverized roots of coltsfoot, licorice root, marshmallow, pansy and anise seed.

The flowers are carefully gathered from July to September, preferably in the morning during dry, sunny weather. The blossoms are directly plucked from their calyces, rapidly dried in an airy place and stored in airtight containers. The roots should be gathered in early spring prior to flowering.

As a household remedy, decoctions of the flowers or roots have been used to alleviate whooping cough, tonsillitis, bronchitis, difficult breathing, mild diarrhoea, vomiting, intestinal cramps, internal injuries, inflammation of the stomach and bladder, and kidney congestion. The roots and flowers can be prepared in hot water and the steam inhaled to alleviate nasal congestion, sore, irritated throats and asthma.

When decoctions of the flowers are added to baths they relieve bedwetting and irritated, inflamed haemorrhoids and skin. The macerated fresh flowers are often infused in warm olive oil and the resulting liquid applied to swellings, bruises, frostbite, inflamed and pustulent inner ear infections and varicose veins. The flowers and leaves are boiled in milk and applied, in fomentations and compresses, to soothe burns, boils, purulent wounds, and eye and skin inflammations, and the flowers can also be boiled in water to yield an excellent skin lotion and hair tonic. The dried leaves can also be smoked in order to cool and soothe dry, sore windpipes and chest congestion.

Mullein was once extensively used as an incense and adornment in churches on holy days. The dry, woolly down of the leaves and stem was used as tinder and lamp wick. For funerals and other occasions, the long stems were coated with tallow to yield a slow-burning candle with an iridescent flame. Mullein was associated with a number of folk traditions. In France, on St John's Eve, great branches of the plant were passed across bonfire flames and the ashes taken home as a protection against thunder. In Germany, young women hung the flowering stems over their beds to ascertain their life span.

Valerian *Valeriana officinalis*

The roots of valerian – or garden heliotrope – are collected in September and October, and when dried exude a camphoraceous odour. They have diuretic, diaphoretic, antispasmodic, astringent properties, and a tranquillizing and sedative effect on the central nervous system. Valerian is effective in treating anxiety and insomnia resulting from nervous conditions. During World War I, valerian was a treatment for shell shock in combatants, and it has been used to cure headaches, dizziness, heart palpitations, migraine, depression and neuralgia. Despite extensive research, none of the plant's individual constituents has been shown to be responsible for its soothing activity. The effectiveness of the crude drug indicates that the calming effect of valerian is a result of the synergistic (coordinated) activity of several principles.

In treating insomnia, valerian may be strengthened with an equal amount of hops, but valerian tea is best prepared in a cold infusion (10–12 hours), as boiling partially destroys valepotriate, an active constituent. Soothing and sleep-inducing effects can be gained by adding valerian extract to baths.

Excessive and prolonged use of valerian may be addictive and result in adverse reactions, so that after 14 days of treatment a temporary shift to lemon balm is advisable. Valerian relaxes the muscles of the gastrointestinal tract, and has been used to treat nervous, cramplike stomach disorders, flatulence, chronic diarrhoea and constipation.

In European herbal medicine, valerian has been used as a vermifuge, an antidote for poison; and to relieve asthma, heavy breathing, stitches in the side, liver congestion, jaundice, spleen and ear ailments and menopausal conditions in women. Combined with lime or linden flowers, valerian infusions were a popular anticonvulsive treatment for epilepsy.

Dried herb

LURE AND INTOXICANT

Valerian is pleasantly intoxicating to cats, who greatly enjoy digging up, rolling in and chewing its roots and leaves. In the Alps the roots are placed in rooms to accustom cats to new surroundings. The scent of valerian was also used to lure rats into traps, and the Pied Piper was supposed to have carried the roots to help him rid the city of Hamlin of this vermin. Valerian is also placed in hives to keep bees close to their nests, and rubbed on earthworms to attract trout to the bait.

Valerian was sacred to the Germanic goddess Herta, who rode a stag, and held a valerian stalk and hop tendrils as reins. Rededicated to St Benedict, valerian was used in pre-modern Europe as a religious incense, condiment, perfume and in England as a pot herb and seasoning. The foetid root was considered a defence against pestilential diseases. Valerian was hung up to ward off demonic beings and lightning, and milk was poured through valerian wreaths to prevent spoilage by witches.

Herbal Healing in the East

Ayurveda is the principal traditional medical system of India, Pakistan, Nepal and Sri Lanka, and has also influenced medicine in Tibet, Burma and Malaysia. Another widely influential Eastern healing system is Chinese traditional medicine, which spread to Korea and Japan and southward into Thailand and adjacent areas, where it is complemented by both Ayurveda and Unani, the traditional Arab medicine used by millions of people in south Asian countries and in all east Asian countries with significant Muslim populations. Unani (from "Ionian") medicine has its roots in the Hippocratic theory of body humours from early Greece. The legacy of the Greco-Arab medical tradition, as expressed in the hot–cold theory of humours, is a pervasive element in popular medicine from Latin America to the Philippines.

There are many smaller, regional medical systems throughout the Orient. For example, Kampo, the healing art of Japan, is still widely used. Oriental medical systems share a holistic approach – which integrates the physical, mental and spiritual – and an emphasis on prevention of illness and strengthening the body's resistance, rather than on curing disease. A common basic concept is that of an underlying life energy – termed *prana* in Sanskrit, *ch'i* in Chinese and *ki* in Japanese – that supports every organism and is united with the life of the universe.

Spiritual health is as important as – and is an integral part of – physical health in Asian medicine. The burning of these purifying juniper leaves by Tibetan pilgrims preserves their health as surely as any diets or medications.

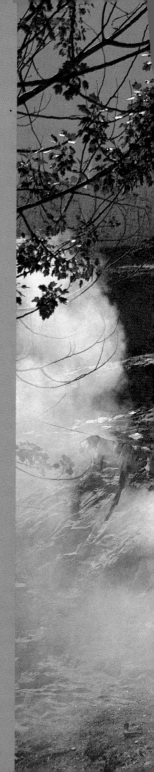

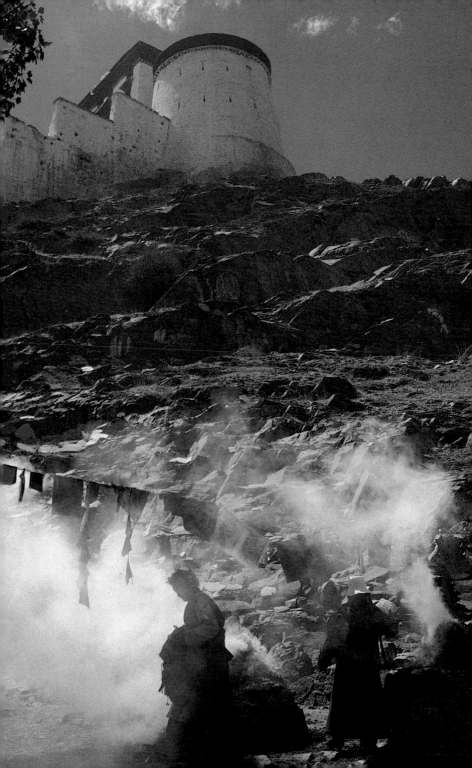

Ayurvedic principles

Ayurveda, or the science of life, is more than a system of medical treatment. It also maintains health by the proper use of dietetics, physical exercise, positive, unselfish thought, fresh air, heat and sunlight. Ayurveda – along with yoga – is integrated into a complex philosophical system called *smakhya*, which does not only deal with human difficulties. As a result, Ayurveda also addresses itself to the diseases of elephants, domestic animals and trees.

According to Ayurveda, the human body comprises three basic elements: *doshas*, *dhatus* and *malas*. The *doshas* regulate the physiological and biochemical activities of the body and its cells. The *dhatus* are the body tissues and the *malas* are the substances used

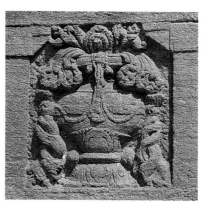

The amrit kalash, *or pot of immortality, here carved on a wall in Vijayanagar in India, is the Ayurvedic symbol of health and longevity.*

by the body and excreted in modified form as waste products. These three elements must maintain a dynamic equilibrium between themselves in order to preserve good health.

The universe is classified into the Five Great Elements: air, water, earth, fire and ether, which are linked to the five senses of the body and their associated organs (the skin, the tongue, the nose, the eyes and the ears, respectively). The Five Elements are the products of energy emerging from a divine cosmic force (*Brahman*). The arrangement of the Five Elements in the body is a microcosm of the universe and Ayurvedic medicine re-establishes harmony between the individual and the life of the universe by balancing universal forces within the patient. The Five Elements are metaphorical categories: each Element actually contains the other four, and it is the most prominent feature of an Element that determines its name. The salient feature of earth is matter; of water, the force of cohesion and attraction; of fire, potential and kinetic energy; of wind, the force of movement and of ether, empty space. In the human body the Five Elements are interpreted in terms of their taste (*rasa*), pairs of attributes (*gunas*), such as hot and cold, or wet and dry, and post-digestive taste (*vipak*).

Ayurveda recognizes seven *dhatus*: plasma and lymph, haemoglobin, muscle tissue, adipose tissue, bone tissue, marrow and nerves, and reproductive tissue. The *dhatus* transform into each other in strict sequence with the aid of a nutrient plasma that arises from the digestive process. Thirteen channels of circulation (*srotas*) transport the nutrient plasma, the *doshas*, to the organs, tissues and systems to maintain them. For the organism to function well, these channels must remain open so that the process of circulation is unimpeded.

Faulty circulation leads to an accumulation of substances in the channels, adverse metabolic reactions and other effects which result in illness. Digestion, absorption, assimilation and metabolism are regulated by biological fire (*agni*). Any imbalance of the *doshas* impedes the working of the biological fires in the tissues and cells, impairing metabolism and bodily resistance and leading to the accumulation of toxic wastes in the body.

EARLY AYURVEDA

The origin of Ayurvedic medicine is shrouded in mystery. Ayurvedic medical texts present divergent mythological accounts of its origins and transmission through a lineage of divine and semi-divine beings. Despite attempts to locate its origin in Vedic texts, Ayurveda was not originally a Hindu priestly (Brahmanic) science. Vedic medicine was dominated by demonic illnesses and magic rituals, and medicine and healers were denigrated and excluded from Brahmanic society.

The ancient Indian physicians found acceptance among communities of renunciants and mendicants (*sramanas*), outside the social order. These wandering monks, primarily Buddhists, developed an empirical medical science from a vast storehouse of medical knowledge which was codified in early Buddhist monasteries, where hospices and infirmaries were established. This medical system was gradually assimilated into the Hindu social, religious and intellectual tradition.

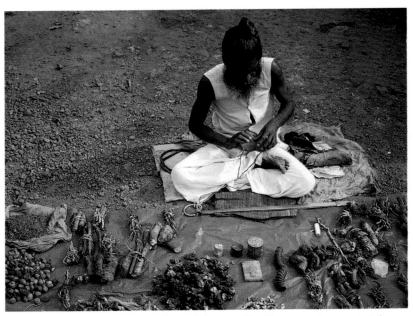

A modern-day wandering herbal sadhu, *or holy man, selling his wares on the streets in India.*

Ayurvedic diagnosis

The *tri-doshas*, which sustain and regulate all organic and mental processes, are composed of the five elements in condensed form. Each *dosha* – wind (*vata*), bile (*pitta*), and phlegm (*kapha*) – is the product of two elements. *Pitta* is made of fire and water, *kapha* is made of earth and water and *vata* is made of air and ether. Although the *doshas* permeate the entire body, they are thought of as belonging primarily to certain regions: *kapha* to the lungs, *pitta* to the stomach and *vata* to the colon.

Vata is the most important of the bodily humours, and regulates all biological and metabolic processes. It flows through all the body passages and plays an active role in the nervous, respiratory and circulatory systems. A deficiency of *vata* therefore results in diseases of the respiratory and circulatory systems, as well as the digestive system. *Vata* is disturbed by physical strain, insomnia and eating the wrong kinds and amounts of food. *Pitta* controls the hormones, enzymes and all metabolic processes. Disturbances of the *pitta* can result in 40 different illnesses, often brought about by anger and aggression, fatigue or a faulty diet. *Kapha* regulates the other two humours, lubricates the moving parts of the body and provides moisture for the brain, eyes and skin. *Kapha* also provides sexual energy and

---

TELL-TALE ORGANS

Diagnosis in Ayurveda is conducted by examining the tongue, pulse, eyes, face, lips and nails. The basis of much diagnosis is that the organs and their ailments can be mapped on to different body parts, as shown in the diagram of the tongue below (this diagram is a mirror-image, commonly used to help in self-diagnosis).

The smaller diagrams show some typical illnesses. In general, a tongue that is whitish indicates problems with *kapha*, one that is yellowish with *pitta* and one that is brownish with *vata*.

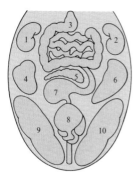

1 Left kidney
2 Right kidney
3 Intestines
4 Spleen
5 Pancreas
6 Liver
7 Stomach
8 Heart
9 Left lung
10 Right lung

sensitive colon

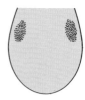

kidney disorder

delicate heart

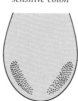

bronchitis (froth)

toxins in colon (white)

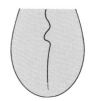

low backache (crooked midline)

The Ayurvedic theory of the *doshas* forms the basis for maintaining health, as well as the diagnosis and treatment of illness. *Dosha* means "trouble" as well as humour, indicating that any kind of disturbance in equilibrium will result in debility and illness. This may involve either an excess or a lack of one or more humours. The degree and kind of imbalance depends upon the constitution of the individual, season of the year, climatic conditions and astrological forces. Hence, Ayurvedic medicine is a form of therapy that is very carefully tailored to the individual. However, in general, *Vata* is aggravated during the summer, *pitta* in late autumn, and *kapha* during the spring, so that special precautions must be taken to ward off diseases caused by these *doshas* during their special seasons.

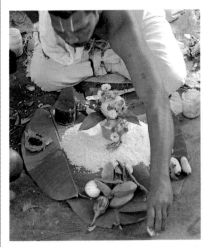

In this ceremony, rice is a healing agent through its symbolic role as "the mother of life".

aids digestion and mental processes. When *kapha* levels drop, through lack of exercise or faulty diet, the results are hardening of the arteries, digestive ailments, stiff joints and anorexia, among other diseases.

The *doshas* manifest themselves in unique combinations which give rise to constitutional body types (*prakruti*). At the moment of conception, an excess of one or two *doshas* will give rise to a

---

ALTERNATIVE HEALING

Ayurvedic medicine suffered a decline during Muslim and colonial rule but returned to prominence on a wave of 20th-century nationalism. However, Western medicine is still widely used in India, particularly by the modern, urban elite.

There are many other healing traditions, such as naturopathy (*prakritis cikitsa*), Unani Tibb (used by the Muslim population) and Siddha (used in Dravidian

areas such as Tamil Nadu). Tibetan medicine (*Emchi*) is popular in northern, frontier regions, such as Sikkim, Ladakh and Darjeeling. In addition, there are diverse forms of traditional medicine among the many indigenous groups (*adivasis*), who possess an enormous repertoire of medicinal plants.

The spiritual disciplines of yoga and tantra also use prescriptions to prevent and cure both somatic and psychosomatic disorders.

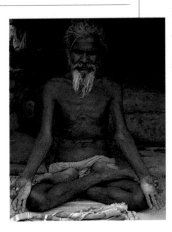

characteristic physical constitution and psychic temperament. The constitutional types are prone to specific disorders and have their own food and drug regimens. Quinine, for example, may be safely administered to a *kapha-prakruti* person, but is harmful for a *pitta-prakruti* person. When someone with a *pitta* constitution has a non-*pitta* type of disease, it will not be serious and can easily be cured.

There are seven constitutional types: pure *vata*, *pitta* and *kapha*; three in which two *doshas* exist in equal strength; and one possessing all three. All *doshas* are simultaneously present in

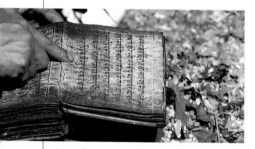

Ayurveda is not restricted to India, and is in fact the most popular traditional system of healing in the neighbouring countries. However, Ayurvedic techniques have become fused with, and modified by, local traditions and beliefs. Here an Ayurvedic practitioner in Kathmandu reads from a text as part of a healing ceremony.

any individual, with subtle variations, but everyone has a tendency to one or more elements. Diagnosis of the individual's constitution is based on twenty aspects, including body frame, skin, appetite, stool, dream motifs and pulse.

Vata-type people are marked by dry skin and hair, thin small boned frames (although they may be tall or short),

and physical underdevelopment. They are creative, active, restless, with high energy but low endurance. Although intelligent and intellectually inclined, their thought is abstract rather than practical. Since their energy occurs in the upper body portion, they are inclined to poor circulation in the lower regions. They tend to suffer from arthritis and lung and nerve diseases.

Pitta-type people are of medium height, frame and weight. They are muscular, athletic, energetic and aggressive. Although they are ambitious, hard working and intelligent, they are often irritable and impatient. They have a capacity for leadership, obsessions and fanaticisms. They are prone to suffer from ulcers and diseases of the blood, intestines and spleen.

Kapha-type people are stocky and heavy-set, but nevertheless are frequently agile and athletic. They are good humoured, emotionally stable, prefer a sedentary life-style, digest their food slowly and like rich, heavy foods. As a result they suffer from heart disease and diseases of the joints, lymph, stomach and lungs.

A susceptibility to certain diseases is indeed statistically linked with different constitutional types. There is a high correlation between the thin, ectomorphic type and a susceptibility to ulcers, tuberculosis and gastrointestinal diseases. Diseases of the gall-bladder and osteoarthritis are associated with a thick, stocky, well-padded build. Tall, thin individuals are most often the victims of valvular heart diseases caused by rheumatic fever and other infectious diseases, while other forms of heart disease are associated with the athletic,

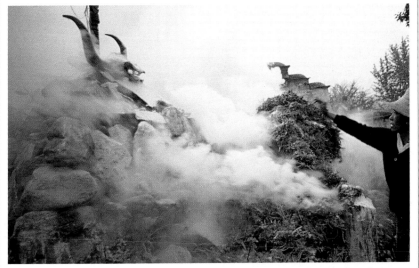

A Tibetan burns juniper leaves to fumigate a shrine, combining ritual and practical purification.

mesomorphic body. Pancreatic diabetes predominately affects stocky, well-padded people, while those with pituitary diabetes fall into tall–thin and intermediate groups.

Ayurvedic treatment consists of the elimination of toxins by means of therapeutic vomiting, purgatives, enemas, blood-letting and nasal administrations of oils, sedatives, powders (such as *gotu kola*), ghee or salts. Any remaining toxins are then neutralized by means of diet, exercise, fresh air and sunlight. It is also considered important to get rid of emotional toxins – negative feelings which can be purged by first being aware of them and then releasing them from the mind. Ayurvedic medicine primarily uses combinations of herbs, each one of which may have a specific action, or all of which may work together synergistically to neutralize toxins.

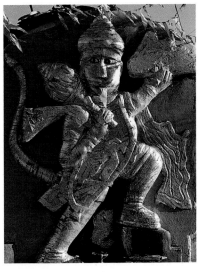

A Rajasthani carving of Hanuman the monkey god bringing humanity the holy mountain on which all the herbs of Ayurveda grow.

AYURVEDIC DIETS

In Ayurveda there is no distinction between foods and medicinal plants. All are classified according to two energies (cold and hot) and six tastes (sweet, sour, salty, pungent, bitter and astringent) which indicate the molecular composition, properties and therapeutic action of a substance.

In general, substances with attributes opposite to those of the *dosha* (see pp.76–8) are used in Ayurvedic therapy. *Vata* people should avoid cold, pungent, bitter, light rough substances and take hot, heavy, smooth, sweet and sour substances. Pungent herbs and sweet nutritious foods, such as ginger, are used to dispel stagnant and deficient *vata* illnesses. *Pitta* persons should avoid hot, acrid, sour, salty, sharp, smooth substances and take cool, bitter, astringent and soft substances. Bitter, dry tonics and diaphoretic herbs dispel *pitta*-related problems such as colds, infections and inflamed skin. Diuretics and purgatives eliminate excess *pitta*. *Kapha* people should avoid cold, bitter, sweet, soft substances and take hot, acrid, pungent, astringent, sour, salty, light and rough substances.

Therapy may include fasting, massage with warm herbal oils and stimulating, mind-clearing herbs, such as guggal and myrrh. The essential energy of the body (*ojas*) may also be strengthened with tonic herbs, such as ashwaganha and shatavari. Amla fruit is used as a rejuvenative tonic, a food, and as a cosmetic. By means of a dynamic equilibrium of tastes, amla stimulates the brain to rebalance the *doshas* within the body. Amla fruit is high in vitamin C and also has antiviral, antibacterial, antioxidizing and cellular regeneration properties.

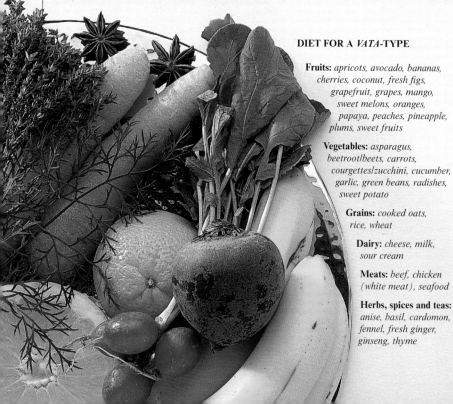

DIET FOR A *VATA*-TYPE

Fruits: *apricots, avocado, bananas, cherries, coconut, fresh figs, grapefruit, grapes, mango, sweet melons, oranges, papaya, peaches, pineapple, plums, sweet fruits*

Vegetables: *asparagus, beetroot/beets, carrots, courgettes/zucchini, cucumber, garlic, green beans, radishes, sweet potato*

Grains: *cooked oats, rice, wheat*

Dairy: *cheese, milk, sour cream*

Meats: *beef, chicken (white meat), seafood*

Herbs, spices and teas: *anise, basil, cardomon, fennel, fresh ginger, ginseng, thyme*

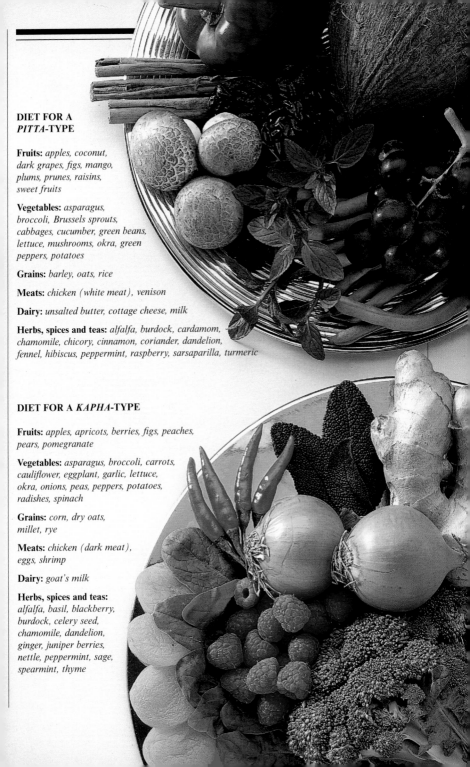

DIET FOR A *PITTA*-TYPE

Fruits: *apples, coconut, dark grapes, figs, mango, plums, prunes, raisins, sweet fruits*

Vegetables: *asparagus, broccoli, Brussels sprouts, cabbages, cucumber, green beans, lettuce, mushrooms, okra, green peppers, potatoes*

Grains: *barley, oats, rice*

Meats: *chicken (white meat), venison*

Dairy: *unsalted butter, cottage cheese, milk*

Herbs, spices and teas: *alfalfa, burdock, cardamom, chamomile, chicory, cinnamon, coriander, dandelion, fennel, hibiscus, peppermint, raspberry, sarsaparilla, turmeric*

DIET FOR A *KAPHA*-TYPE

Fruits: *apples, apricots, berries, figs, peaches, pears, pomegranate*

Vegetables: *asparagus, broccoli, carrots, cauliflower, eggplant, garlic, lettuce, okra, onions, peas, peppers, potatoes, radishes, spinach*

Grains: *corn, dry oats, millet, rye*

Meats: *chicken (dark meat), eggs, shrimp*

Dairy: *goat's milk*

Herbs, spices and teas: *alfalfa, basil, blackberry, burdock, celery seed, chamomile, dandelion, ginger, juniper berries, nettle, peppermint, sage, spearmint, thyme*

The Chinese healing of harmony

Chinese medicine is an extremely complex and sophisticated healing system which emphasizes prevention of disease using tonics and substances to heighten the resistance of the body and its immune system. Medicinal plants are only part of the healing process, in conjunction with diet, massage, physical and deep breathing exercises, and a salutary life-style. Chinese physicians also examine the patient's emotions, social relationships, work habits and environment.

The Chinese symbol for yin and yang captures the way in which these two relative principles control, balance and transform into each other to produce movement and energy.

Good health is a function of maintaining harmony with the ceaseless, cyclical patterns of transformation and change which permeate the universe. Emanating from an ultimate, undefinable force (*Tao*), movement and energy are manifestations of, and are given a definite structure by, the interplay between the active, fertilizing principle of yin and the reactive, materializing principle of yang. The individual is a spatial and temporal mirror of the universe, and external things are functions of the living organism. Diseases are the results of both internal (biological and psychic) and

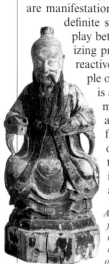

A 16th-century polychrome figure of Lao Tzu, the original Taoist master, who is often credited as the father of Chinese medicine.

external (social, diurnal, seasonal and cosmic) functions. Illness is a blockage of the flow of yin and yang.

Foods, herbs, body types and organs, stages of disease and therapeutic techniques have been grouped with events, attributes and substances of every kind according to a yin–yang binary system of classification. However, Chinese physicians went further by developing a vast system of correspondences and associations using a series of elementary principles. For example, one set of guidelines used to ascertain therapeutic effects and the body's reaction to plant substances is the four energies – cold, hot, warm and cool. Pungent, sweet foods produce warm or hot sensations in the body. Sour, bitter, salty foods impart cold or cooling sensations. Herbs with warm (yang) properties dispel internal cold and warm the stomach and spleen. Hot and warm substances are used to treat cold diseases and symptoms, such as poor appetite, pallidness and weak limbs. Cold or cool herbs soothe the nerves and have antibiotic and sedative effects on diseases of an inflammatory, hypermetabolic nature. Therapy also relates to the constitution of the individual. Someone with a cold physical constitution needs foods with a hot or warm energy. A hot physical constitution calls for cold foods. The four energies and other elementary principles are integrated into a more precise and complex interlocking system known as the five elements (*we-hsing*).

PRESCRIPTIONS

Chinese herbology is the most developed form of ethnopharmacology in the world. Although there are thousands of Chinese formulas, the basic repertory consists of 120 prescriptions, each containing six to twelve substances. A medicinal plant is classified according to its essence, action, direction and contracting or dispersing effects. Ginseng, for example, is classified as warm, tonifying, moistening, ascending and contracting.

Pills, powders and medicinal soups may include substances with similar actions, combined to heighten therapeutic effect, or two constituents with

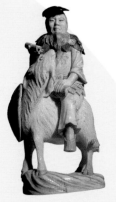

A 19th-century ivory carving of Shen Nung, an emperor-god of herbs and medicine.

opposing actions which are combined to inhibit each other's actions or neutralize toxicity. Combinations are designed to lead constituents to a pathological site and to fit specific organ imbalances.

For example, sweet–warm combinations, such as ginseng and astragalus, are used to treat low heart *ch'i* (see p.85) and blood, stomach and spleen deficiencies; bitter–sweet combinations (gentian and liquorice) remove heat from the intestines and bitter–warm combinations (magnolia and immature orange) regulate the flow of stagnant *ch'i*.

In Chinese dietetics, food plants act on specific organs. For example, celery is beneficial for the stomach and liver and leek for the heart. Foods of various flavours, energies and action are consumed, since overconsumption of one kind may strengthen one organ but weaken others.

ENERGY FLOW

Chinese medicine discovered smallpox immunization and the circulation of blood long before Western medicine, but it is not primarily concerned with anatomical knowledge. Chinese medicine concentrates on the dynamic relationships of body regions and the energy that flows through them, rather than individual organ-functioning. Therapy also focuses on the (yin) body surfaces, where the exchange of *ch'i* energy (see p.85) between the (yang) interior and the outer world takes place.

Chinese physiology maps the flow of *ch'i* along a defined pathway of twelve

channels or meridians connecting the limbic system (seat of the emotions), head and visceral organs. There are also eight irregular channels that function as a reservoir of *ch'i* energy. When the body organs are in balance, *ch'i* flows smoothly. When the organs are excessively contracted or expanded the flow of *ch'i* is impeded. Herbs are prescribed which re-establish the flow, tonify the basal *ch'i* and expel pathogens. Once the *ch'i* energy is flowing again, health can be restored by the body's own self-healing mechanism.

A modern acupuncture chart, showing the flow of ch'i.

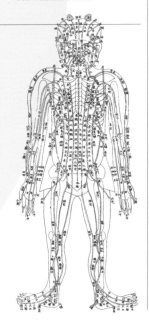

Elements, flavours and directions

Taste is a guiding principle for healing and maintaining balance in the overall system of Chinese herbalism. Each of the five flavours – sweet, sour, pungent, bitter and salty – manifests its own pharmacological action and helps to determine the function of a medicinal substance. A sixth flavour, bland or tasteless, is sometimes subsumed under sweet and has diuretic properties.

Flavours are usually used in combination. For example, a pungent–sweet combination, such as fresh ginger and liquorice, is used to correct disturbances of the nutritive and protective *ch'i* (energy). Sweet-flavoured herbs and foods strengthen the stomach and spleen, and have warming, soothing and nourishing properties. (However, excess sweets result in diarrhoea, chronic constipation, or excessive urination.) Complementing the properties of sweet foods, pungent substances are

beneficial to the large intestines. They promote energy and blood circulation, induce perspiration, increase metabolism and have warming, dispersing and drying properties. Pungent foods, such as peppers, onions, mustard and cinnamon, are also used to prevent and treat cold (yin) respiratory diseases, such as sinus conditions, asthma and emphysema. However, taken in excess they cause diarrhoea and faulty breathing. Some individual herbs already have a mixture of flavours, and dodder, for example, is both sweet and pungent.

Sour, astringent substances are used to tonify and regulate the effects of other foods. They also promote digestion and help eliminate toxins from the blood although, in excess, they prevent the liver from eliminating waste. Bitter substances act on the heart and small intestine to improve circulation and digestion.

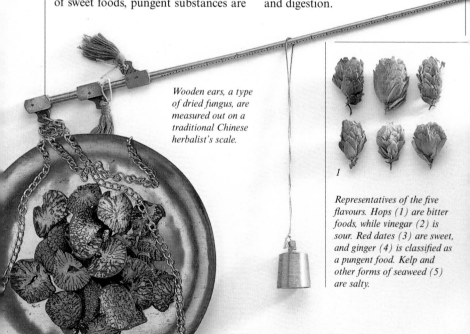

Wooden ears, a type of dried fungus, are measured out on a traditional Chinese herbalist's scale.

1

Representatives of the five flavours. Hops (1) are bitter foods, while vinegar (2) is sour. Red dates (3) are sweet, and ginger (4) is classified as a pungent food. Kelp and other forms of seaweed (5) are salty.

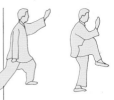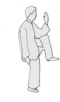

In excess, bitter foods cause heart palpitations and irregular intestinal functioning. Bitter foods, such as radish leaves, reduce body heat and dry body fluids. Moderate amounts of salty foods, such as barley, are beneficial to the kidney and bladder but in excess raise the blood pressure by constricting the kidneys. Salty drugs dispel water, relieve constipation and soften hard tumours. Saltiness travels in the blood, so people who suffer from circulatory and heart ailments should refrain from eating salty foods.

In addition to their energies (see p.82) and flavours, drugs, foods and diseases are also classified according to their direction of movement: ascending, descending, floating (or outward) and sinking or inward. Coughs and vomit rise, sweat moves outward, constipation moves inward and diarrhoea moves downward. Drugs having an opposite

THE NATURE OF *CH'I*

Ch'i is a form of emotional potential energy. Since it is simultaneously connected to a person's unconscious and physiological functions it is not reducible to either the mind or body and cannot be accounted for within the framework of mind–body dualism. It circulates within the body while at the same time intermingling with the *ch'i* energy that is present in the social and physical environment. Although the underlying nature of *ch'i* is unknown, its external manifestations have been described as resembling a form of electromagnetic energy. Chinese healing modifies *ch'i* through many techniques, including herbalism, acupuncture and the exercises called *Tai ch'i chuan* (above).

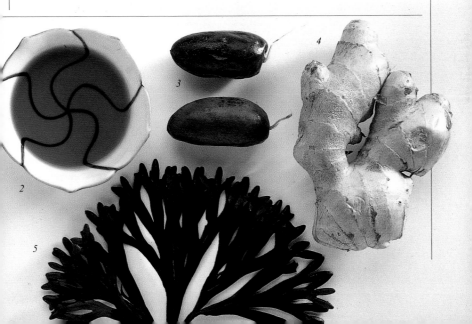

direction to that of the disease are used as cures. Warm, hot, pungent, sweet foods and drugs move upward or outward. Cold, cool, sour, bitter substances move downward or inward. Some medicines have two or more directions. Kudzu, for example, first descends, then rises, and ginseng is effective in treating both high and low blood pressure because it moves in several different directions. The nature of the medicine to be prescribed is further specified by the disease site and the season. Cold, bitter, salty foods that move inward should be taken during the winter. Sweet, pungent foods that move outward are taken during the summer and sweet, bitter foods that move upward are taken in the spring.

Medicinal plants are also classified according to the vital meridian or channel they affect (see pp.82–3). Because a

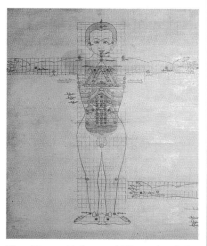

The widespread influence of Chinese thought is shown by the similarity between ch'i *diagrams and this 18th-century medical tanka, a teaching aid used in Tibetan medicine.*

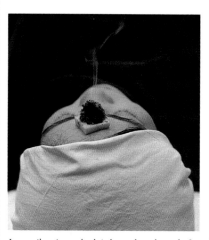

In moxibustion, a herb is burned on the end of an acupuncture needle, on a pad placed on the skin or in a stick held just above the skin. Its healing powers radiate to the ch'i *meridians.*

herb's pharmacological action may encompass different organs, it can affect various channels at the same time. Radish seeds, for example, act upon the spleen, stomach and lung channels by dispersing stagnant food and causing lung *ch'i* to dispel any built-up phlegm. Certain herbs, such as bletilla and kudzu, serve to direct the other herbal constituents of a prescription into a particular channel and its related organs.

The ability of herbs to affect a whole meridian means that parts of the body not considered by Chinese medicine to have vital organs can nevertheless be treated. A pain at the front of the head, for example, can be treated by herbs with an affinity for the stomach, because the stomach meridian passes up through the face and forehead.

FIVE PHASES OF TRANSFORMATION

The five elements or phases is a complex mnemonic and metaphorical device used by Chinese doctors to correlate complex sets of relationships between therapeutic treatments, bodily organs, symptoms, secretions, emotions, colours, tastes, odours, foods, chronological processes and the physical environment. Each of the five elements – wood, fire, earth, metal, water – possesses its own particular set of correspondences, which is used by Chinese physicians along with pulse measurements, dreams and the history of the patient in making a diagnosis.

The five elements connect the colour and flavour of a drug to body organs. For example, the combination white–pungent–metal is related to the large intestines and yellow–sweet–earth influences the stomach. Each pair of elemental organs is nourished by specific foods, while other foods are destructive to this organ group. Choosing foods and herbs appropriate to the season ensures the unimpeded circulation of *ch'i* and adapts the life of the individual to that of the macrocosm. The clockwise flow of the circle forms the *Shen* or vital principle cycle. Each phase of an element nourishes the organs within that element and passes *ch'i* on to the next phase. Thus, the element earth provides

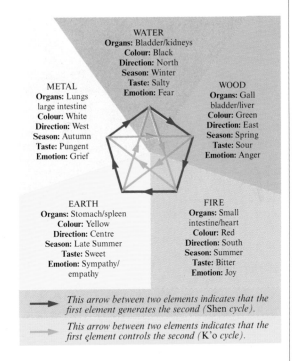

WATER
Organs: Bladder/kidneys
Colour: Black
Direction: North
Season: Winter
Taste: Salty
Emotion: Fear

METAL
Organs: Lungs large intestine
Colour: White
Direction: West
Season: Autumn
Taste: Pungent
Emotion: Grief

WOOD
Organs: Gall bladder/liver
Colour: Green
Direction: East
Season: Spring
Taste: Sour
Emotion: Anger

EARTH
Organs: Stomach/spleen
Colour: Yellow
Direction: Centre
Season: Late Summer
Taste: Sweet
Emotion: Sympathy/ empathy

FIRE
Organs: Small intestine/heart
Colour: Red
Direction: South
Season: Summer
Taste: Bitter
Emotion: Joy

*This arrow between two elements indicates that the first element generates the second (*Shen* cycle).*

*This arrow between two elements indicates that the first element controls the second (*K'o* cycle).*

ch'i to the stomach and spleen and then passes *ch'i* on to the lungs and large intestines (metal).

The *K'o* or control cycle specifies the antagonistic and destructive relationships between the elements and their organs. Water controls fire, so that deficient kidney energy (water) can result in high blood pressure and heart palpitations (fire). The kidneys are controlled by the stomach and spleen (earth), so that an imbalance in the spleen due to excessive sweet and sour foods will obstruct the flow of kidney *ch'i* (water). An excess of yang in earth may stem from an

imbalance in wood via the *Shen* cycle or a deficiency in metal via the *K'o* cycle. Herbs are administered which reduce the energy of earth or add energy to metal.

In medicating an element system, the previous organs in the *Shen* cycle are also treated. In order to strengthen the spleen (earth), the small intestine energy (fire) should also be healed. An imbalance during the season associated with one element will lead to an imbalance in the season of the next. For example, weakness in the spleen during the late summer will appear as a lung disorder in autumn.

Popular Chinese herbs

Chinese plants are becoming increasingly used in the West. Of those shown here, five exhibit striking medicinal and disease-preventive properties.

The mo-er or black tree mushroom (*Uricularia polytricha*) is used as a longevity tonic and for painful menstruation. Also known as the tree ear or wood ear mushroom, it contains adenosine and other blood-thinning compounds which prevent strokes and heart attacks. Mo-er compounds also stimulate the immune system and retard cancer in animals. The shiitake mushroom (*Lentiuns edodes*) contains compounds which lower blood cholesterol levels and, block the effects of highly saturated fats. Shiitake also contains lentinan, which stimulates the immune system to produce interferon, a powerful anti-viral and cancer-killing substance.

Ginkgo (*Ginkgo biloba*) is used in Chinese medicine to treat pulmonary and heart diseases, and to regulate urine emission. It expands the blood vessels, increases circulation, especially in deep-lying arteries, and prevents the blood from clotting. Ginkgo extracts are widely used in Europe to improve metabolism in the brain and to prevent oxidative damage to the cerebral membranes. Ginkgo constituents

1 Star anise
2 Ginkgo nuts
3 Da xue teng
4 Jing jie
5 Xanthium fruit
6 Tea
7 Huang lian
8 Shiitake mushroom
9 Dang-gui
10 Sweetgum fruit
11 Safflower
12 Black tree mushroom

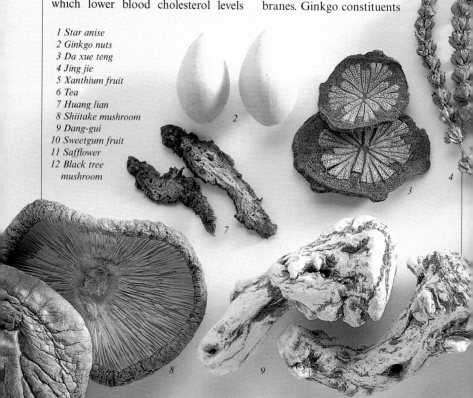

improve cerebral capillary flow and are used to treat sleep disturbances, depression and symptoms of cerebral insufficiency in the elderly.

Dang-gui (*Angelica sinensis*) is used in Chinese medicine to harmonize *ch'i* energy, increase coronary circulation, and reduce arterial blood pressure. It also has anti-inflammatory, pain-reducing and tranquillizing effects on the cerebral nerves, and is used in treating irregular or difficult menstruation, PMS, menopausal symptoms and postpartum debility.

Black tea is a popular stimulant, which is also effective in treating diarrhoea. Unlike black and oolong tea, green tea is heated with dry air or steam, which prevents its cancer-fight-

ing catechins from oxidizing. Drinking green tea reduces the risk of cancer. The Japanese, who drink a lot of green tea show low rates of all types of cancer, especially stomach cancer.

The other herbs are all used in varying amounts in Chinese prescriptions. Star anise is a stimulant and diuretic, which promotes the flow of milk in new mothers. Jing jie promotes sweating and reduces swellings and abscesses. Xanthium fruit and sweetgum fruit both expel wind and dampness and are effective against rheumatic pains. Huang lian is a mild sedative and antitoxin which eliminates heat and dampness. Safflower and da xue teng both improve the circulation of blood, and da xue teng also purges blood toxins.

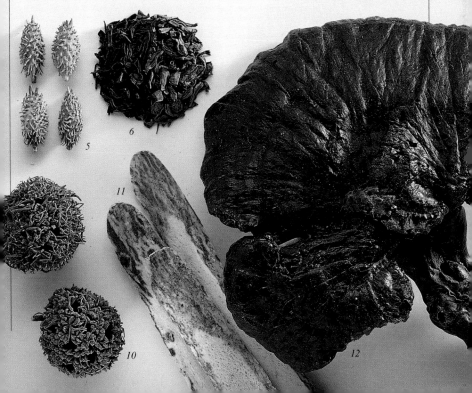

5
6
11
10
12

Thailand

The traditional Thai medical system was introduced by Buddhist monks who established monastic hospitals there some 800 years ago. Thai medical theory contains the Ayurvedic *tri-dosha* humoral system (see pp.76–9), but uniquely adapted to Thai culture. The presence of several regional variants of Thai traditional medicine and the professional secrecy of the practitioners greatly contribute to the rich diversity of Thai herbal practices.

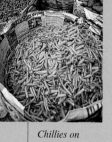

In rural villages, each household has a repository of herbs. Medical knowledge is transmitted within a family, and also by means of formal apprenticeship to a traditional practitioner. In urban centres, the medical system was once transmitted through the royal courts and the monasteries, but is now state regulated. Traditional practitioners are trained in an official school with an authorized syllabus and licensing examinations.

Chillies on sale in a Thai Chinatown market.

Thai medicine is based upon thousands of different prescriptions or formulas written on long concertina-like strips of pleated paper, kept in homes, temples and royal libraries. Each written formula lists a disease, its symptoms, the plant ingredients for a cure, their weight, mode of preparation and administration. Only natural ingredients are used in a cure, and the prescriptions are continuously updated and submitted for official approval. Although Thai herbalists commonly possess hundreds of written formulas, only the most effective prescriptions are used in daily practice.

Illness is generally thought to be the result of an elemental imbalance caused by sudden changes in climate, psychosocial stress, or the overexertion of physical and mental energies. Illness can be caused by an excessive intake of sweet or fatty foods, an unbalanced diet of only fish or meat, or by consuming hot foods when the body is overheated. Other factors include the patient's age and place of residence, and the time when the illness occurred, which can all make the body less able to withstand

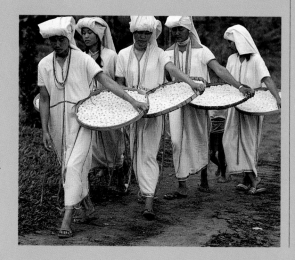

Girls of the Karen tribe carrying chrysanthemums which will be made into tea.

THE DEADLY POPPY

Opium is extensively grown among the poor ethnic populations of northern Thailand as a cash crop and for its analgesic properties. It is extremely addictive, and in detoxification centres a Hmong shamanic ritual has been incorporated into the treatment in order to bolster the patients' motivation and increase their involvement in the programme. This ritual is based on the Hmong opium-creation myth.

At the beginning of Hmong time, there was a king whose daughter, although beautiful, suffered from a foul body odour. Because no one would marry her, she vowed to avenge herself by making magic that could not be lifted. Upon her burial, her breasts became the poppies that yield opium milk and her vagina became

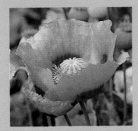

Opium is derived from the poppy Papaver somniferum.

the tobacco plant. The opium goddess is believed to visit the male opium smoker in his narcotic dreams, and eventually possesses him. In an Akah variant of the myth, a beautiful woman had many suitors but only seven gained her affection. In order to avoid discord, she made love to all of them, although she knew it would kill her.

In the shamanic ritual to aid withdrawal from opium dependence, the goddess is persuaded to leave the

addict's body to take up residence in a miniature palace that has been built for her. A basket is richly decorated with a clay model of the goddess, figurines of her entourage and domestic animals. The addict's opium pipes and utensils are also put into the palace. After invoking the deities to witness the addict's sacred vow never to use opium again, the shaman petitions the goddess to move to her new abode.

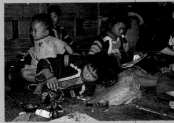

Opium addicts from the Lahu of northern Thailand.

the presence of germs and influence the development of the disease.

Bodily balance is restored by changing the amounts of heating and cooling substances ingested. Medicinal plants and combinations, bodily reactions and some illnesses are classified as hot, neutral and cold. Although the *dosha* model serves as a general reference point, it is not systematically linked to the selection and use of medicinal plants. Rather, medical theory is linked to therapeutic practice in terms of nine medicinal tastes. Sour taste, for example, indicates anti-mucus activity and astringent-tasting plants are used to

heal wounds and, internally, for treating colic, diarrhoea and other stomach disorders. Thai medicinal plants may be ingested with foods or applied with massages. They can be prepared in teas or infusions, poultices, washes, juices, steam baths and as inhalants. Emphasis is placed on a smoothly-functioning digestive system and the Thais are avid consumers of herbal tonic drinks before coming home from work and on other occasions. The Thai *materia medica* of some 700 plants includes aloe, banana, basil, garlic, ginger, guava, lemon grass, lime, pineapple, pumpkin, sugar cane and tamarind.

Regional Traditions

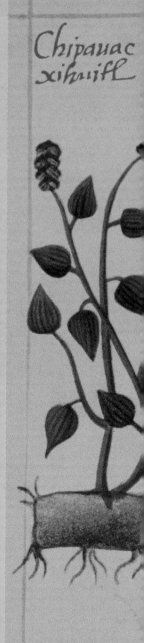

Herbal traditions are open and dynamic systems, constantly changing in response to historical and environmental conditions. One factor in this process is the continuous exchange of medicinal plants between the various regions of the world. Plants whose origins can be traced back to classical European antiquity are used today by Andean herders and Pacific islanders. Similarly, many Oriental or exotic plants, such as aloe, gingko and ginseng, are avidly used by Europeans. Both the continuity and the differences between the various traditions can be seen in the ways in which plants are prepared for use.

Although infusions and poultices are universal, there is a notable difference between, for example, the African use of dried, powdered plants and the Polynesian preference for freshly extracted plant juices. However, both Africans and Native North Americans use warm cornmeal poultices to treat boils and pustules. The Cherokee method of asking the spirit of the plant for an appropriate remedy is echoed in the close relationship that Amazonian healers have with plant spirits. The spirit of religious dedication with which herbalists worldwide go about their work is, in fact, perhaps the most striking similarity between them.

A page from the 16th-century Central American Codex Badianus, *showing the influence of new medicinal plants on old European practice. These herbs are listed as a cure for "vomica", a term used by the Roman writer, Pliny, to refer to boils.*

Domica

Africa

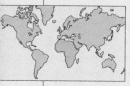

The diversity of cultures, ethnic groups and botanical regions in Africa means that it is extremely difficult to make any generalizations about healing strategies. Excluding the Ethiopian, Egyptian and Arabic medical traditions, which are based upon written records, there are some 1,000 cultural and linguistic groups in Africa, each having its distinct mode of healing. Almost 90 percent of the population resides in rural areas and relies, to a greater or lesser extent, on traditional forms of healing. Realizing that the rural populations cannot be completely provided with capital-intensive, high-technology medicine in the foreseeable future, government and international organizations make a concerted effort to evaluate and incorporate traditional medicine into the primary health care system.

There is great variety and fluidity in the roles and practices of native African doctors. While some only cure with plants, others combine herbal remedies, to a greater or lesser degree, with divination as diagnosis (as practised by the Zambian healer, right), surgery, scarification, bone-setting, blood letting and other practices. Recourse is made to household remedies, or the recommendations of neighbours or a local herbalist if the illness is considered minor and due to natural causes. If no relief is obtained the patient proceeds to a diviner, who has greater diagnostic and therapeutic ability to cure with complicated techniques of purification and sacrifice. Or, as among the Bafulero of Central Africa, the sick first consult a diviner who, on the basis of a diagnostic interview and divination, then directs patients to a herbalist, surgeon, midwife or medical clinic.

The African pharmacopoeia is rich with cures for many diseases, but African flora is imperfectly known pharmacologically, and only a few of its

ZULU HEALING

Medicines that treat illnesses caused by mystical agents, such as sorcery and ancestral spirits, are classified by the

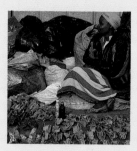

Zulu medicines for sale in Natal, South Africa.

Zulus as black, red and white. They are administered ritually by professional practitioners and re-establish the balance between a person and the environment, which was disturbed by sorcery or pollution. Mainly prepared from bark and roots, they may also contain ingredients from wild animals. They are always taken in the sequence, black, red and white, although either black or red may be omitted.

Black medicine is a drastic, potent remedy which expels evil. White medicine may be a sedative or tonic which works off the effects of the black medicine and restores the

patient to a state of complete wholeness. Red medicine, symbolic of twilight, is an intermediate remedy in the process by which the patient is taken out of the darkness by black medicines and into life and daylight by white medicines. Representing rebirth, it is administered during the transitional state when the patient is neither sick nor healthy.

Heat denotes sickness, while health is associated with coolness. White is "cool" and black and red "hot", so black and red medicines are always heated and white medicines are taken uncooked or raw.

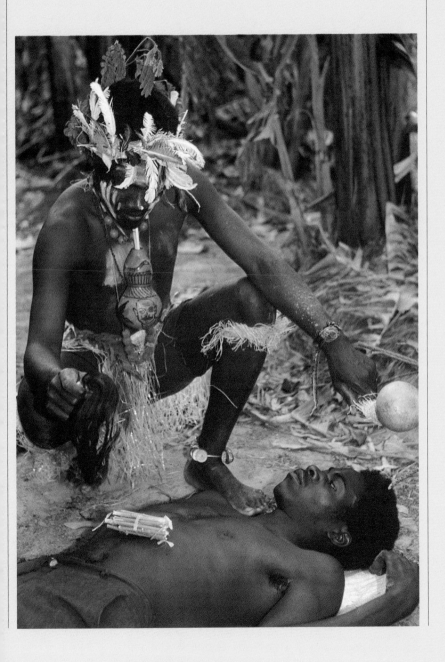

plants, including the anti-carcinogenic periwinkle, have been incorporated into modern medicine. Physostigmine derived from the Calabar bean, a West African ordeal poison, is used internationally to treat glaucoma, anti-cholinergic toxicity (affecting the nerve fibres) and Alzheimer's disease. *Rauvolfia vomitoria* is used by West African native doctors for prolonged sleep therapy and as an initial treatment for acutely disturbed mental patients, often to make them more amenable to psychosocial therapy. This *Rauvolfia* species contains reserpine and ajmaline, which are used in modern medicine to treat high blood pressure and anxiety.

Healing in Africa is concerned with the restoration or preservation of human vitality and the harmonious

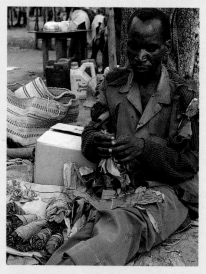

The Meru have several kinds of medical practitioners, including mwaanga *(shown here) who cure solely with medicinal plants.*

working of the universe. Illness is subsumed under a broader category of affliction, which implies a disruption of the symmetrical, moral order through which the self is connected to the social group, environment, ancestors, spirits and the cosmological order. Consequently, rational and magical notions of the causes of disease come into play simultaneously and are not clearly distinguished from each other.

In some groups, such as the Thonga of southeastern Africa, training is minimal and transmitted by heredity. Individuals are taught to specialize in the preparation of medicines for a particular type of illness. More common, however, is training from 3–20 years as an apprentice to an expert herbalist or priest. The novice, a male, is taken into the forest to learn the names, descriptions and uses of the plant medicines. Since the apprentice is also learning how to harness spiritual forces, he must remain celibate and follow numerous other regulations during his training period. If, on the day of graduation, divination indicates that he has broken any of these regulations, he must make a sacrifice, pay a fine and be retrained for 3 more years.

The Meru herbalists of northern Tanzania do not have the complex system of medicines with magical powers commonly present in African medical systems. They do not pray or carry out ritual and divinatory actions in their practice or while collecting plants, and they have reworked their concept of disease-causing worms to accomodate the theory of invisible germs. However, Meru herbalists do receive some knowledge of medicinal plants from their

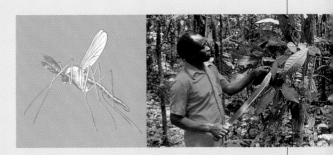

Malaria, transmitted by anopheline mosquitoes (right), is one of the more prevalent infectious diseases in Africa. Most districts have their own remedies. The Meru use Achyranthes aspera, *which is also one of their five remedies for heartburn. In Cameroon, the remedy is* Lavigeria macrocarpia *(far right).*

supreme deity in dreams. Diagnosis is based on an interview with the patient about his or her subjective experiences or symptoms, and observations of physical signs, such as bloody diarrhoea. Symptoms and causes are clearly differentiated by Meru herbalists, and a remedy is chosen on the basis of both.

Meru herbalists have several remedies, varying in potency, for each ailment. The selection of the remedy and dosage is based upon the age and sex of the patient, his or her individual peculiarities and the strength of the particular substances being used. The concern for detailed and stable dosages, say the herbalists, distinguishes them from nonprofessional hawkers of herbal medicines. Diseases are attributed to environmental conditions (cold, heat, rain, dirt), eating habits, personal hygiene (such as eating with dirty hands), worms, social disorder, poisoning, sorcery, the condition of the blood, ancestral spirits (which cause blindness and mental disturbances) and God (who sends epilepsy and leprosy). One Meru herbalist practises 56 cures for the digestive system alone, directed against five types of diseases, with one particular stomach disease having thirty-one separate remedies.

SCARS AND SALVES

Many African herbal medicines are not taken orally. By covering a patient's head with a blanket, boiling mixtures of herbs can be used as inhalations for colds, fevers, chest complaints and mental disturbances. Enemas are also widely used to treat abdominal pain and painful menstruation.

In powdered form, plants may be used for sniffing to induce sneezing and cure headaches, or taken dry on the tongue. Dried roots are burned to ashes and mixed with oil, which is rubbed into fine linear incisions made in the skin over sprains and other painful areas.

For non-localized pain, leaves are soaked in water and used to cover the sick person's body. Boiled leaves are placed on body parts as a means of applying heat. When they cool they are reboiled. This treatment can last for half an hour every morning and evening for 3 weeks.

Heated herbal pastes are applied to open wounds, ulcers and to ease rheumatic pain and aching feet. A hot corn porridge is applied to boils to aid the formation of pus, and hot applications of peppers are used in bone setting. In making ointments, roots are powdered and added to a tree-sap which is then boiled in a little water. This greasy salve is used to soften the skin.

The South Pacific

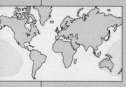

The various island chains of Polynesia are relatively isolated from each other, and have developed their own distinctive set of medical concepts and practices. Between them, they use some 400 different medicinal plants. During the 20th century, many plants have acquired new uses, with some being dropped from the Polynesian pharmacopoeia and others, previously not used, added to it.

Polynesian herbalists may be general practitioners or specialists who treat one or more types of disease. Polynesian herbalism is focused on the treatment of childhood ailments and infant delivery, so most herbalists are women, although in Hawaii there are both male and female practitioners. In addition, there are male bone-setters, massagists and specialists in treating illnesses caused by ancestral spirits.

Herbalists acquire their skills in 1–7 years, starting in childhood, in an informal manner from a family member. Additional expertise is acquired from other healers, from ancestral shades through dreams, or by experimentation. The knowledge to diagnose and treat illnesses is believed to be spiritually endowed and medicinal efficacy is imparted to the plants by the power of the healer. Herbal remedies are family possessions. If used by others, without family approval, the plant would lose its powers. Polynesian herbalists accept no money for their services, since doing so would dissipate their healing powers. Although they do accept small gifts, their major gratification is the ability to help others and the prestige obtained from doing so.

For severe or life-threatening diseases, Polynesians utilize the services of hospitals and clinics, although in the Cook Islands traditional practitioners are also consulted for the treatment of cancer and tuberculosis. Traumatic injuries, fractures, digestive ailments and other minor illnesses are treated by herbalists and other folk practitioners. In some islands almost all families have a member who is medically proficient. These healers always use fresh bark, flower buds, leaves and rhizomes, never

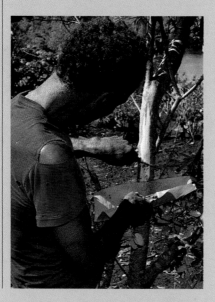

Medicinal plants are grown in gardens or gathered in the wild. While some plants require no rituals when gathering them, others must, in order to be effective, be gathered ritually. In collecting bark from certain trees on Tonga, the bark is scraped from the side facing the rising sun while from other trees the west side is used.

AUSTRALIA

Although traditional Aborigine healing has been largely replaced by Western methods, medicinal plants are still used, especially in northern Australia when synthetic medicines are ineffective. (A chestnut shrub, *Castanospermum australe*, the bark of which was used as a native poison, exhibits pronounced activity against the HIV virus.) Australian Aborigines recognize a variation in plant potency according to season and geography, and different clans use different medicinal plants, or the same plants may be used in different ways from clan to clan. Women practise herbal medicine, while difficult surgical procedures and healing by means of the invocation of spirits are mainly in the hands of men of high degree, or shamans. On Groote Island all adults have knowledge of plant medicines, with the women treating other women and children, and the men treating other men.

Medicinal plants are prepared fresh daily and frequently compounded with

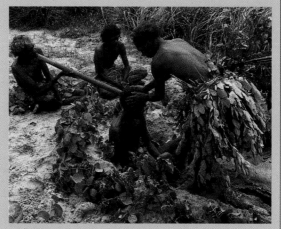

To treat burns, wounds, cuts and bites, the sap of gum trees is applied, or boiled and used as a wash. Chewed leaves are directly applied or crushed leaves may be soaked in water and the liquid poured on to the wounds. Heated leaves are pressed on to control bleeding, and bark is made into a pad and bound over the injury.

animal and insect parts. Of the thirty-five medicinal plants used by the Alawa people of northern Australia, 44 percent are used to treat skin ailments and the rest for intestinal, respiratory and other ailments. For coughs and colds, plant juices or leaves soaked in water are ingested. Leaves and twigs are steeped in hot water and

Australian Aborigines consider the various species of native fuchsia, or emu bush, to be their most important and sacred plants. Eighteen species of the genus are used medicinally. The Alyawarra of central Australia alone use seven for colds and flu, headaches and chest pains, fever, diarrhoea and wounds, among other ailments.

the vapour inhaled, or boiled and the liquid patted on the chest. Inhalation is also used against headaches. To treat diarrhoea, leaves or taproots are eaten raw, or a liquid infusion is rubbed on the stomach or drunk.

In the desert of central and northern Australia a peculiar multi-purpose body-smoking method of healing is used. The patient stands or squats over a hole filled with smouldering, leafy branches. Alternatively, to treat vertigo and nervous conditions, hot coals are placed in the bottom of a trench and covered with the leaves and branches of the wattle tree. The patient is laid on the branches and covered with more leaves, resulting in profuse sweating.

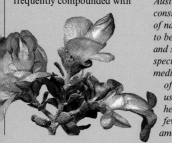

dried. Tree bark is pounded and the other parts are chewed or mashed in a bowl. The macerated material is then folded in a piece of cloth, dipped into water or coconut water and squeezed to extract the juices. Medicinal plants are rarely boiled, and most are applied externally, although some may be taken internally at the same time. In some eastern Polynesian islands, such as Tahiti and Hawaii, purgatives are taken as a preventive medicine, for digestive problems and to rid the body of toxic substances. In Hawaii, single plant remedies or simples are preferred, whereas in other islands combinations of up to forty ingredients are utilized.

Dietary restrictions are an essential component of Polynesian herbal therapy, and an emphasis is placed on cleanliness and frequent bathing. If a herbal treatment is not effective, the patient is sent to a clinic or to a curer specializing in diseases caused by ancestral spirits, which are native illnesses and cannot be cured by Western medicines. Family spirits are roused by abuse, aggression and treachery within the family, as well as by infractions of behavioural rules (*tapu*). These spirits cause a family member to become afflicted with possession or a chronic illness not amenable to regular therapy. A cure may involve eyedrops, baths and massages made with basil or other strong-smelling plants noxious to the spirits, which will drive them away. In some cases, the healer will go into a trance in which the spirit explains the reason for the illness. An emotional and cathartic way to treat spiritual illnesses is with an assembly of the family members, who publicly confess and forgive their mutual wrongdoings.

Massage is a highly developed method of healing in Polynesia, used to treat fractures, muscular strains, displaced or malfunctioning organs, and to set bones. Massaging is also used to move back the life essence, which is said to wander from its proper location, the upper abdomen, to other body parts, resulting in illness. Plant remedies used in massaging are made with coconut oil, or rubbed on the skin after an initial application of coconut oil.

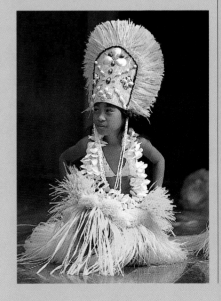

In Hawaii, plants used in treating internal ailments are collected with the right hand and plants for treating external injuries are picked with the left hand. Children in Hawaii are sent to gather plants since they are considered pure and undefiled. This child is also a hula dancer. Originally, the hula was a fertility dance performed by dancers wearing leis, *or symbolic garlands of interwoven flowers.*

The white-flowered bottle gourd, Lagenaria siceraria, *is widely used as a laxative and purgative, to treat body pains, skin blotches and mental disturbances due to sleeplessness. It once assumed a key role in Polynesian material culture, being used to fabricate masks, bottles, bowls, syringes, fishing equipment and musical instruments. Bottle gourd fragments have been found in Peruvian sites dated at 13,000BC, although the plant is thought to originate in Africa. The bottle gourd seems to have been one of the first plants ever cultivated.*

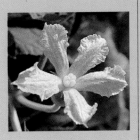

THE PACIFIC DRUG

The drinking of kava, an infusion of the roots of the shrub, *Piper methysticum*, is central to Polynesian social and ceremonial life. The physiological effects of

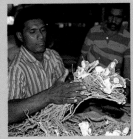

Kava roots in a Fijian market.

drinking kava are a tranquil, friendly state of well-being, followed by a profound, dreamless sleep with no morning-after grogginess. Being a spinal rather than a cerebral depressant, kava does not impair mental alertness. Taken too freely and frequently, strong kava can cause ataxia, liver and kidney dysfunction, blood abnormalities, eye problems, weight loss and scaly ulcerations of the skin.

Kava is served on all social occasions, such as political gatherings, marriages, funerals, and secular feasts and parties. As a symbol of peace and friendship, it is used to establish and cement friendly relations. In western Polynesia and Fiji, kava is served in a public ceremony abounding in elaborate rules of etiquette. The participants are seated in circles around the presiding chief in gradations of rank reflecting their genealogical seniority. The kava is prepared by young women or men who chew the subterranean stems and roots into a pulp which is deposited in bowls, stirred, and then strained through a fibre sieve. This mastication releases and emulsifies the resin in the cellular tissue, resulting in a stronger brew.

The assembly is served the resinous liquid in strict order of rank. Through the power or *mana* of kava the presiding chief and other participants are brought into contact with the sacred, and temporarily incarnate the ancestral deities, blurring the sacral and profane worlds. The speeches delivered in kava ceremonies are eloquent and very detailed, containing terms of respect known only to the nobility.

The chemical constituents of kava have analgesic, anti-convulsant and muscle-relaxant properties, and are useful in the treatment of various skin diseases. Pacific island peoples have long employed the drug to treat fever, skin infections, urogenital inflammations, gonorrhoea, centipede bites and other ailments. Today it is also served in urban kava bars and has become a drug of abuse among Australian Aborigines, who take kava resin with petrol and alcohol to synergistically increase the drug's effects in the brain.

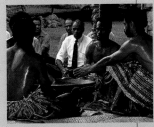

The kava ceremony under-scores the hierarchy as well as the unity of social life.

North America

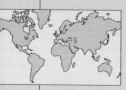

European interest in the subject of North American medicinal plants dates back to 1535, when the crew of Jacques Cartier's scurvy-stricken ship was healed by Native Americans who administered decoctions made from the needles of hemlock (*Tsuga canadensis*). Two hundred years later, James Lind, a British naval surgeon, read an account of Cartier's experiences, and initiated the experiments which eventually proved the dietary basis of scurvy.

A common North American plant, Joe Pye weed (*Eupatorium purpureum*) received its name from a Mohegan, Joseph Pye, who taught settlers in 1787 how to use the plant to cure typhoid fever. The stem of this plant was also used by the Cherokee as a form of natural pipette, to spray medicines into the urethra, on fractured limbs and other afflicted body parts.

One of the earliest published pharmacopoeias, or standardized drug lists, was compiled in 1787 by Johann Schoepf, the surgeon general of the Hessian army in the American War of Independence. It contained a description of 335 medicinal plants, most of indigenous origin. Sixty of these Native American medicinal plants, which had been adopted by settlers, were later added to the official United States pharmacopoeia.

The early settlers were constantly on the alert for new drugs and before long plants such as May apple root, sassafras, sumac, ginseng, rattlesnake root and pinkroot were being exported on a large scale to Europe. The Virginia snake root (*Aristolochia serpentaria*) was so highly valued by the Cherokee that they placed an embargo on its

SECRET SOCIETIES

Specialized medicinal plant knowledge was often the property of curing guilds or societies, such as the Iroquois False Face Society. These sodalities carried out group shamanic practices in conjunction with the use of medicinal plants, directed toward propitiating the spiritual agent believed to be responsible for an illness. On special occasions, these societies performed great healing or "life- [vitality-] giving" ceremonies, which abounded in songs, prayers, ritual and drama, and extended over periods ranging from a few hours to 9 days.

The Ojibwa Midewiwin or Grand Medicine Society had four kinds of medical practitioners, only one of whom specialized in herbal medicines. Medical knowledge was learned in four stages, from lower to higher. Herbalists were considered at the lowest stage and received most of their plant remedies at the time of their initiation.

This mask was used in False Face Society ceremonies to help appease the spirits.

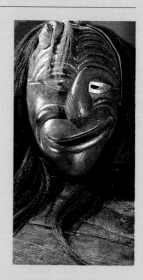

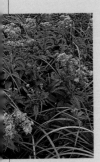

Joe Pye weed.

export, and imposed the death penalty on anyone found carrying the roots from their territory.

Among a number of groups, such as the Penobscot, medical plant knowledge was common property, and not restricted to a few individuals. However, in many groups, such as the Salish, certain individuals, commonly women and the elderly, were especially familiar with medicinal plants and their uses. Almost every Plains woman possessed knowledge of certain plants, the medicinal properties of which she alone knew. Among the Algonkin of Virginia, medicinal plant knowledge was widespread but priestly doctors were consulted in greater emergencies. These individuals were held in great esteem and kept their herbal knowledge a secret except for some remedies, such as for snake bites, which were needed immediately. Herbal knowledge was learned and passed down from the priest-healer to his successor, within the family, or to apprentices and friends. Among certain groups, the inheritance of herbal knowledge was passed through alternating sexes or given to maternal nephews every second generation.

Since a high value was placed on plant knowledge, the medicinal usages of a plant and the songs used while gathering and administering it may

have had to be purchased. Among the Forest Potawatami the fee paid to effect a cure entitled the purchaser to a knowledge of the plants used and how to prepare them. This wisdom could not be divulged by the buyer to anyone without receiving the same fee. Knowledge of plant medicines could not be transmitted even to a family member without compensation, since the information would not otherwise be treated with proper respect.

Among the Omaha, medical treatment was specialized, with one person curing fever, another haemorrhages, and so on. Sioux medicine men usually

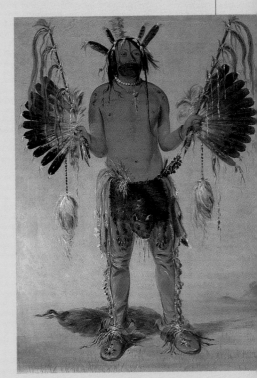

Old Bear, a Plains medicine man painted by George Catlin in 1832.

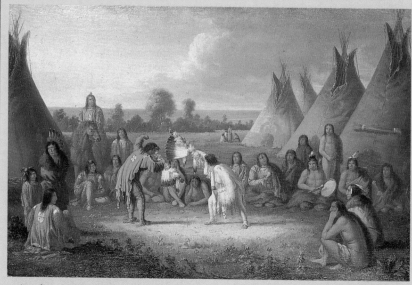

A medicine pipe stem dance, painted by Paul Kane in the mid-19th century. Pipes were integral to Native American ceremonies, and their tobacco smoke carried prayers to the great spirit.

treated one particular disease and treated it successfully. They would not try to treat all diseases for they could not expect to succeed in all cases.

Medicinal knowledge was acquired by accident as well as by experiment. Californian Cahuilla shamans and herbalists tested various treatments and learned the precise dosage of plant substances that would effect cures. Medicinal plants were experimented with cautiously and in sparing amounts before being introduced into general use: a plant which produced an astringent effect when put in the mouth was thought to produce the same effect on the stomach when swallowed. Should an experimental plant provide relief or otherwise prove helpful, it would then be developed into a common remedy.

Throughout North America, medicinal plants had to be collected at the right time of the year to produce the best results. For some plants the proper season for gathering was a very short period of 3–4 days. The leaves of a plant would be gathered early in the morning when the plant was in flower. Roots were gathered at the close of the growing season or before the beginning of spring growth. For certain herbal mixtures the plant species had to be picked in a prescribed order.

The Montagnais believed that bark from a tree trunk or plant stem had to be pulled downward, never upward, in order for it to be efficacious. The Cherokee and other southeastern tribes always took the bark from the eastern side of a plant and when roots were taken it was necessary to collect the ones that ran toward the east. The sun's rays, it was maintained, purified the side they touched and rendered those parts bitter and more powerful. If the Mohegans obtained a medicine by scraping a plant upward from the stem, it was used as an emetic; if scraped downward, it was used as a cathartic. The Delaware dipped water from a downstream current for emetics and against the current for cathartics.

The medicine bag of one Iroquois herbalist contained prickly ash, sassafras root bark, Rhamnus cathartics, calamus rhizomes, wintergreen hemlock needles, pussy willow root and blackberry root. The medicine bag shown here is stuffed only with weasel skins, which Crow women took out and danced with to ensure the fertility of the sacred tobacco.

Before gathering a plant, a prayer or song was recited and a small gift of tobacco was offered to the spirit world and the power dwelling in the healing herb, invoking it to become curatively active. Before gathering a plant, Cherokee medicine men faced the four cardinal directions reciting a formula, or circled the plant either one or four times, reciting prayers during their revolutions. After pulling the plant out of the ground by the roots, a sacred coloured seed (*Lithospermum canescens*) was placed in the hole as a

ANIMAL WISDOM

Knowledge of medicinal plants was often received in dreams from animals. The bear was considered the chief of all animals in regard to medicinal plants since it was the only animal that dug up roots, and ate the same nuts and berries that were used in making medicines.

In one legend a Blackfoot woman who was ill with tuberculosis noticed some beaver tracks and left some food for the animal, which returned the favour by appearing in a dream-vision to give her a cure for her illness. She tried the remedy – an infusion of lodge pole pine resin – while uttering a special song. After much

vomiting, her chest cleared. Pine was used by several North American groups to treat pulmonary complaints, tuberculosis, rheumatism, wounds and ulcers.

The herbal knowledge that was received in dreams was not accepted unthinkingly, but was subjected to practical tests of its effectiveness, and judged accordingly.

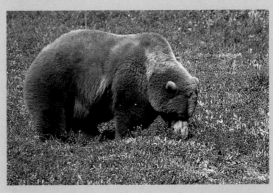

The North American brown bear is especially zealous in digging up roots, nuts and berries while preparing for its winter sleep.

compensation to the Earth for the plants taken from her. There were individual rituals for the preparation of the medicine, its proper care and its administrations. Certain ceremonies were connected with the sowing of medicinal plants. A typical procedure was the planting of seed, the building of a hedge of green branches around the seed-bed, a visit to the sweat house, followed by a cold bath and a solemn smoke, and ending with a feast. To the Crow, the tobacco plant was sacred; it was almost invariably used on solemn occasions accompanied by invocations to their deities. Tobacco was ceremonially used to aid in disease or misfortune, to ward off danger, to bring good fortune, to assist one in need, and to allay fear.

After being used, plant remains were never carelessly thrown away but were preserved about the house. Roots and herbs were usually stored in bags or tied in bits of cloth, ready for steeping. In

PRESERVING THE TRADITION

Among the Cherokee, the sick were taken to community houses where they remained under the care of doctors until they had recovered. Cherokee doctors knew the habitats, flowering periods, medicinal properties and lore of 150–200 different plants, as well as the characteristics of 230 diseases, classified according to the Cherokee worldview. There were about 600 curing formulas, which were recited or sung while the patient was being treated. The invention, in 1819, of an 80-character syllabary by the Cherokee, Sequoya, allowed the formulas to be put in writing.

The sacred formulas of the Cherokee offer a complete description of Cherokee medico-religious and herbal practice. The most important formulas are those used in the treatment of rheumatism. The patient was placed under dietary restrictions and treated with eel oil and ferns. Rheumatism was believed to be caused by the revengeful spirits of slain deer or by the measuring-worm. To remove rheumatism inflicted by the spirit-owner of the

A contemporary painting of Sequoya.

deer, the wolf and dog – powerful animal spirits and enemies of the deer – are invoked in the curing song.

According to a Cherokee myth, the animals were outraged by the callous brutality of mankind, and exacted revenge by each inflicting a particular disease (Native Americans were, in fact, affected by tularemia and other infectious and parasitic wildlife diseases). The plants held a council and resolved to present the Cherokee with remedies

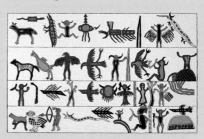

The picture writing of the Ojibwa, in which they recorded myths about the origins of disease.

for all the diseases inflicted upon them by the animals. Hence, for every disease brought about by the animals, there is a remedy in the plant world. Ginseng plants were sacred, and used as an analgesic, anti-rheumatic, a gastrointestinal aid and a tonic. Ginseng was also held in high esteen by the Ojibwas, and was thought to be of divine origin.

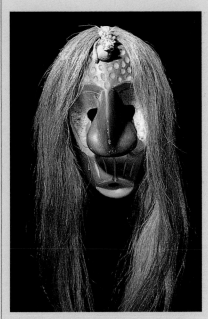

This Iroquois mask was used to treat smallpox. The bundle of tobacco on the forehead was thought to make it especially potent.

groups, even in ecologically uniform areas, such as the southeast. The pre-Columbian North Americans were on the whole a healthy people, and aside from the effects of intertribal warfare, they had few diseases, so there was no demand for a large variety of medicines. Common ailments were treated with medicinal plants, but sweating, massage, prescribed diets, scarification (see p.97), cupping and moxibustion (see p.86), bleeding, bone-setting, surgery, and suction to draw out pain were also utilized. Some of the more important medicinal plants used in the eastern woodlands were astringents and fever-reducing agents (dogwood bark, sassafras, sweet gum, yellow poplar), cathartics (*Euphorbia* species, blue flag, May apple root, butternut bark), de-wormers (pinkroot), emetics (puccoon, button snakeroot). Sweat-inducers and emetics were used to treat fevers and an emetic followed by a cathartic was a general treatment for various internal disorders.

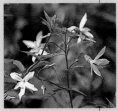

Native American peoples were especially noted for their skill in treating wounds (with *Indian physic was widely used throughout North America as an emetic.*

more southerly climes and traditions, plants were collected on the day of use, except for herbs pertaining to childbirth, which were stored for the winter. Members of the Midewiwin society kept their plants in special pouches, which were never opened without first performing a vapour-bath ritual. If the bag had become wet on a journey, or if for any reason it was suspected that the plants were injured, the individual took a vapour-bath and gave a feast during which the bag was inspected.

Plant medicines varied widely among the 300 groups of Native Americans north of Mexico, and there was considerable diversity in plant usage between green elm bark, powders to cause suppuration or drying, and frequent washes), bruises, fractures and dislocations. Burns were treated with basswood bark and young pine, insect stings with goldenrod, and frostbite with beech and pine resin. An enema syringe, made of an animal bladder and a hollow bird or animal bone, was widely used to treat constipation, diarrhoea, haemorrhoids and wounds. Beaten sassafras bark was placed on putrid ulcers and warm poultices of cornmeal were put on boils, which were later lanced. Poultices of powdered slippery elm bark were utilized for burns, inflammations, wounds and ulcers, and oil from hickory nuts and butternuts was used in liniments for stiff joints.

Venomous snake bites were an ever-present danger for which thirty-five separate cures were known and used in different areas. Many of the plant remedies for snake bite also cause reddening of the skin, the most prominent ones being black cohosh, button snakeroot, Seneca snakeroot, Virginia snakeroot and the white ash.

In diagnosing an illness, Central Algonkian herbalists took the patient's pulse, observed the pupils of the eyes, the condition of the tongue and complexion, felt the body temperature and enquired about the location and nature of the pain. After leaving an offering of tobacco with a prayer to shed light on the disease at a rock shrine, the curer took dream-inducing medicine and went to sleep. In a dream the curer's guardian spirit revealed which herbs and preparations were needed. Plants were thought to be the hairs of the head of Grandmother Earth, so the herbalist chanted her a song while gathering the plants, asking her to impart her power to the medicine. Although some groups, such as the Cherokee, primarily used only one medicinal plant at a time, Central Algonkian herbalists utilized a "shotgun" prescription of between nine and twenty plants. The efficacy of

PLAINS MEDICINE

The purple coneflower (*Echinacea angustifolia*) and related species were the most extensively used medicinal plants of the Plains Native Americans. The peoples of the Great Plains used the root of the plant as a painkiller, as well as to treat a number of ailments, including colds, coughs, wounds, sore throats and snake-bites.

Recent scientific research in Europe has shown the chemical constituents to have anti-carcinogenic, antibiotic, anti-inflammatory and beneficial wound-healing effects. In addition, *Echinacea* contains molecules that stimulate the immune system.

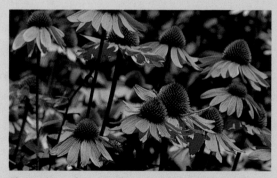

The purple coneflower is still extensively harvested by the Plains Lakota people for a variety of medicinal uses.

The plant or its derivatives may be used to treat any chronic or acute infection which is accompanied by short-term immune deficiency or dysfunction.

Echinacea-derived preparations are currently among the most popular medicines used in Europe and the United States to ward off colds and flu.

plants was ranked, with some being more powerful than others, and the number of plants in a combination represented increasing strength. In applying the remedy, the herbalist recited songs to inspire faith in the patient that health would be restored. Copious draughts of herbal teas were prescribed several times a day, and if the patient had not recovered in 4–8 days, the curer sought further inspiration in a dream and tried a different medication.

Native Americans still use plant medicines to a certain extent, often when modern medicines have failed. The Algonkian Cree currently use more plants for medicines than for food or any other traditional use.

BATHING AND PURGING

Native Americans believed that cleanliness and purity of body were powerful aids to prayer, and that regular purification of the body bestowed immunity from disease. Washing, bathing, fasting and impregnating the lungs and body pores with medicinal and aromatic herbs carried by the steam of the sweat lodge, followed by a cold plunge bath, provided healthy, tonic effects.

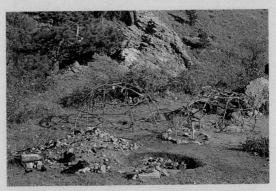

Pole frames are covered with skins to make sweat lodges. At the centre are fire pits for heating stones, on which water is sprinkled.

Emetics and purgatives were often taken as a means of internal purification, and one of the most prominent plants used for the purpose was cassine or yaupon (*Ilex vomitaria*). This evergreen shrub or small tree grows near salt water from Virginia to the Colorado river. Having a high caffeine content, a decoction of the toasted leaves was taken as a stimulating, social beverage throughout the southeastern United States. When boiled for a long time a strong decoction of the plant served as an emetic. Southeastern peoples induced vomiting when they were ill, before critical or hazardous undertakings, before going to and after returning from war, before playing a ball game and before holding a council.

At the annual New Fire or Green Corn ceremony they took copious amounts of

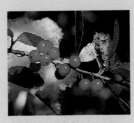

Cassine, which fruits in winter.

cassine, which made them vomit freely. They continued drinking and ejecting for 1–2 days until they had ritually purified themselves. Southern peoples had several methods of preparing cassine for differing strengths, and added other ingredients, such as the button snakeroot, blue flag, rattlesnake fern and paw paw, to impart further strong emetic properties to the mixture. When allowed to ferment and taken in great amounts, cassine induced a trance-like state which enabled communication with the spirit world.

Central America

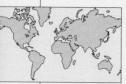

Mexico possesses a rich treasury of medicinal plants because of the great diversity of climates, terrain and ethnic groups. There are 56 Indian-speaking groups and twelve vegetation zones, ranging from alpine scrub to tropical rainforests. About 15–20 million Mexicans use traditional medicine through the services of 180,000 practitioners, who are not legally regulated and supervised.

The use of medicinal plants in modern Mexican life has ancient origins. Medical botany in pre-Hispanic Mexico had reached a high degree of sophistication. Herbal medicine was practised by experienced doctors, surgeons and nurses in hospitals established by the Aztec government. In Tenochtitlàn, the Aztec capital, there were also herb vendors in the markets and apothecary stores. The Aztec nobility dispatched envoys to distant parts in search of new medicinal plants which were brought home, the roots packed in balls of earth and wrapped in woven mantles. In the gardens of Montezuma, the Aztec king, an organized group of physicians performed systematic experiments with these plants and attended the illnesses and "fatigue of those administering government and discharging public affairs". Commoners rarely came to these court physicians for medical aid, because of the expense. However, the medicinal properties of many herbs were common knowledge, and remedies could be obtained from household gardens.

With the fall of the Aztec kingdom to the Spanish in the 16th century, folk practitioners continued to practise in obscurity, while the forty different kinds of Aztec physicians and priests were eradicated. Since then indigenous

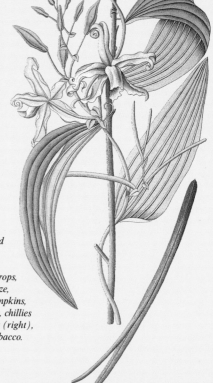

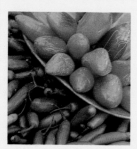

Mexican farmers discovered and cultivated hundreds of present-day crops, including maize, tomatoes, pumpkins, squash, beans, chillies (left), vanilla (right), cotton and tobacco.

MATERIA MEDICA

The Spaniards brought the best known Indian physicians to the College of the Holy Cross on the outskirts of Mexico City to pass on their knowledge of native herbs. One of these teachers, Martin de la Cruz, compiled the first *materia medica* in the Americas in 1552. Known as the *Badianus* manuscript, it was first written in Nahuatl, the language of the Aztecs, and then translated into Latin by Juan Badianus, a native reader in Latin at the College. The herbal gives the Aztec uses of 185 medicinal plants, with 200 illustrations.

Hernan Cortés, the conqueror of Mexico, had his battle wounds healed by his Indian allies, and his quick recovery gave him such a high regard for the native plant doctors that he asked the Spanish Crown not to allow European medical doctors to come to New Spain because they simply could not match the native physicians. The Spanish Crown was anxious to obtain this Aztec medical knowledge, and in 1571 the king sent his personal physician, Francisco Hernandez, to study the medicinal plants of New Spain. In 7 years of work, Hernandez recorded detailed descriptions of 3,076 plants, of which 1,200 included their

medicinal properties. Some of these herbs were quickly adopted by Europeans, and the botanical works of Cesalpino, L'Ecluse and others reflect the introduction of Mexican medicinal plants into the European pharmacopoeia, including senna, scammony, jalapa, vanilla, sarsaparilla, and pimento or allspice. Capsicum or chilli peppers, which were used medicinally by the Maya, yield capsaicin, currently applied in a cream to relieve arthritic pain and

inflammation. The papaya is still used to treat rashes, ulcers and post-operative transplant infections.

Interest has recently been reawakened in the Aztec sweet herb (*Lippia dulcis*) which contains a chemical, hernandulcin, a thousand times as sweet as sugar. Conversely, many plants introduced by the Spaniards, such as chamomile, peppermint, borage, rosemary, feverfew and basil, are now an integral part of Mexican herbal medicine.

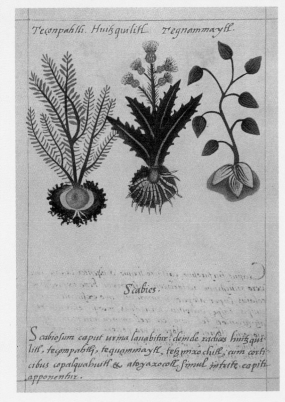

Plants, whose identification is uncertain, listed in Badianus as cures for scabies.

curanderas or curers have been the target of persecution and ridicule. Because indigenous medicine was closely linked to the native religions, Indian curers were considered as agents of the devil, and even the use and administration of medicinal plants were legally prosecuted during the colonial period.

The banning of hygienic and medical procedures such as daily bathing, circumcision and the native vapour bath, which killed syphilitic spirochetes and other microbes, contributed to the spread of disease and epidemic infections. The opposition to native curers took on a new form when, during the 1930s, the village *curandera* was portrayed in national campaigns as impeding the life-saving work of government health employees and thus causing needless deaths. There are regions where campaigns of harassment against traditional medical practitioners continue to this day. The general attitude of physicians toward traditional medicine is that of condescending indifference if not outright contempt. However, since modern medicine is essentially urban-based, the ranks of herbalists, midwives, bonesetters, massagists and healers will continue to be a culturally-relevant and readily available resource for the rural populations.

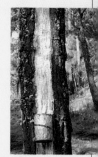

Pine is used by Mexican herbalists to treat sharp pains such as toothache.

According to Mexican herbal medicine, good health involves maintaining an equilibrium internally, interpersonally and in relation to nature and the spiritual world. Body states, foods, illnesses and medicinal plants are classified according to a "hot" and "cold" opposition. An imbalance may be brought about by strong emotional states such as anger and fear, irregular eating habits, overwork, undue exertion and sudden shifts in body temperature.

The herbal tea taken for chills must have warming properties and for a fever the tea must have cold properties, and remedies are always applied in moderate amounts. Particular plants are specified for particular illnesses, and not for general hot or cold diseases. Nor are

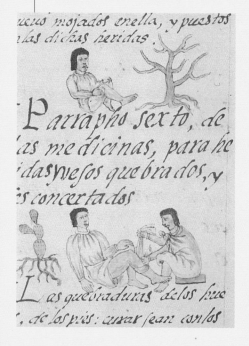

Scenes of everyday curing with herbs, from the 16th-century Florentine codex.

HEALING BREWS

Teas are made from a wide variety of plants. A standard remedy for bile and liver ailments is to drink a cup of fennel tea every morning for 2 weeks. Mints, verbenas and other plants possessing aromatic essential oils and alkaloids are important sources of decoctions and infusions. The leaves of *Salvia* species are used to alleviate stomach distress and aid digestion, and the leaves of orange and lime trees are also used for upset stomachs. Euphorbias are well-known sedatives and purgatives and are used to treat diarrhoea. Eucalyptus leaves in boiling water are used as an inhalant for colds.

One of the most important plants to expel worms is epazote or wormwood, which is also a popular food flavouring. Chilli peppers, which are rich in vitamins, are another popular ingredient in worm expellents and are also used as a laxative. The fruit and extracts are employed in poultices and hot plasters; but if misused may produce serious skin burns. (*Cassia* species are also used in poultices for sores and ulcers of the skin.) The juice of the raw chilli induces perspiration in the treatment of colds and hangovers.

Tagetes lucida, or cempoasuchil, is favoured as an emetic, stimulant, insecticide and for gastrointestinal and pulmonary ailments and is also used in commemorating the dead. It was once pulverized and administered to Aztec captives to diminish their capacity for pain before they were sacrificed.

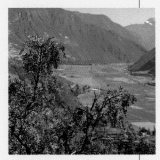

Plants are not only used in the preparations of herbal medicines. In ritual cleansings of the sick, branches of rue, the firecracker bush, the pepper tree (above) or the sweet marigold are used to stroke the body. Although many different curative properties are attributed to herbs, in certain instances they are only effective in combination with prayers and rituals performed when the herbs are being given.

hot and cold considered to be thermal qualities, but are innate and remain unchanged when exposed to changes in temperature. There is individual and regional variation in assigning hot–cold distinctions, but plants are broadly classed according to their smell, taste, colour and habitat. Any plant that is sharp to the taste, such as pine, is considered to be hot. Plants with a bitter taste are neutral. If the leaf feels hot on the forehead the plant is cold; if nothing is felt it is hot or neutral.

In all Mexican towns and cities there are market and store vendors who not only sell herbs but also prepare plant mixtures on the basis of symptoms described by their customers. Many villages have one or more herbalists, who acquired their knowledge and experience from their parents or by means of several years of apprenticeship to an accomplished herbalist. When a family member becomes ill, in most rural areas household remedies are initially used, particularly if the illness is not a serious one. If these treatments are ineffective, recourse is made to a shaman-curer. The illness is then treated as the result of an imbalance between the individual and supernatural entities, resulting from sorcery, soul loss or moral transgressions, such as aggression and non-fulfilment of ritual obligations.

South America

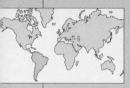

The Amazon Basin is one of the richest regions for plant life in the world. There are some 75,000 species of plants of which only a fraction are known botanically or pharmacologically. The peoples of the Amazon have learned many uses for the plants around them, including the treatment of third-degree burns without scarring, relieving the pain of osteoarthritis, and preventing women from conceiving.

Local people utilize several types of resources when faced with illness, ranging from clinics and hospitals to a variety of herbalists, massagists, spiritists, bonesetters, shamans and home treatments. Both men and women are knowledgeable about the medical uses of wild and cultivated plants, but specialists in herbal healing – usually women – are called upon when the expertise of family and neighbours is insufficient to affect a cure. Midwives also retain special herbal knowledge, especially concerning plants used in childbirth, pre- and postnatal care and infant illnesses. The most common diseases present in the region – gastrointestinal disorders, respiratory ailments, rheumatism, wounds and sprains – are treated with sweat baths, poultices and herbal potions, according to the nature and severity of the illness.

Teas and infusions have always played a major medicinal, as well as social, role throughout South America. This 18th-century Argentinian silver cup and strainer is used for drinking maté, *an infusion of a species of holly.*

Herbal knowledge is transmitted in small groups, through face-to-face interactions, although some remedies are given to curers by spirits in dreams and visions. The mother spirits of the various plants are like people and can be contacted and befriended. When medicinal plants are gathered, prayers are offered to the spirit of the healing plant, invoking her to do battle with the spirits of disease. Cultivated plants have less healing power than wild plants, since they are separated from Nature, the reservoir of spiritual power.

Certain plant species, of which there are over thirty in the Peruvian Amazon, are thought to be benevolent teachers. After taking a purge of the sanango tree (*Tabernaemontana* species), a person will see the mother spirit in a dream, enquiring why the purge was taken. The individual will usually be seeking a cure for an illness, and the mother spirit will give prescriptions to be followed.

Native healers or shamans communicate with plant spirits to ascertain the cause of an illness and to receive remedies. Each shaman has a special relationship with a particular plant, the most important being ayahuasca (*Banisteriopsis* species). In order to be cured, the patient must take the herbal medicine, undergo a strict dietary regimen stipulated by the plant mother and be sexually, socially and spatially isolated. In taking the herbal remedy, the patient absorbs the body of the plant spirit and by following the elaborate dietary prescriptions the patient replicates the behaviour of the plant mother and regains equilibrium by becoming one with her. If the vigorous cure that is stipulated by the plant mother is not

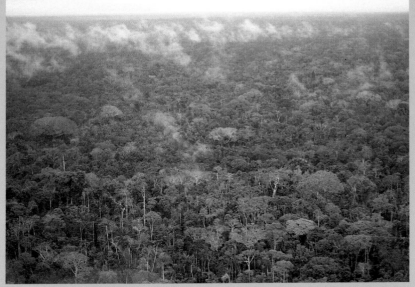

The Amazon Basin in Brazil. The River Amazon rises in the Andes only 100 miles (160km) from the Pacific Ocean, and empties into the Atlantic. The vast surrounding rainforest and its flora are still hardly explored, and thousands of new plants, and new medicines, await discovery.

followed, she will discontinue the cure and may attack the patient, resulting in illness and death.

Early travellers to South America were astonished not just by the number of medicinal plants used by the inhabitants but by the fact that they always used one plant at a time in affecting their cures, rather than combinations of several plants. Despite the increasing influence of modern medicine, plants continue to play a major role in the diverse medical systems of South America. In all urban centres vendors sell, diagnose and prescribe medicinal herbs in public markets. In Bolivia, vendors who dispense and prescribe herbs in urban markets are even organized into guilds. In many South American cities the sale of medicinal plants is a million-dollar business and in the main market of La Paz, the Bolivian capital, there are over 130 herbal vendors. In addition, a diverse array of urban *curanderos*, often located in the poorer neighbourhoods, treat a wide variety of complaints using medicinal plants.

As a synthesis of European, Indian and African traditions, urban herbalism exhibits enormous diversity in the plants, diagnostic and therapeutic methods used. Knowledge of medicinal plants is, however, less extensive than among rural and Indian populations. Among the Mapuche of Chile and Argentina, most men and women have knowledge of more than 250 medicinal plants. The Yupa of Venezuela are also renowned for their knowledge of medicinal plants. Any Yupa man or woman can name and describe hundreds of plants and their utility.

Among the Yaruro of Venezuela, practical knowledge of medicinal plants is based upon an accumulation of empirically verified observations of symptoms and treatments. Symptoms such as vertigo, anaemia, diffuse pain, coughs and fevers are linked to particular organs of the body and, in diagnosis, eye colour, complexion, stools, saliva, urine and the subjective sensations of disease are attentively observed. However, Yaruro medicine, like that of all other South American indigenous peoples, is a manifestation of a religion which permeates all individual and social behaviour, morality, feasts and other institutions.

Among the Warao of the Orinoco Basin, female herbalists treat natural diseases caused by toxic gases, poor blood, body malfunction, over-exertion and exposure to the elements, but epidemic diseases and psychiatric disorders are attributed to mystical pathogens and are treated by male shamans. The Mbyá-Guarani of Paraguay possess 198 medicinal plants and numerous therapeutic

Snuff has always been one of the most popular plant preparations in South America. This 500-year-old silver tube (left) was used by the Incas for taking snuff. A modern-day Matses from Peru has the hallucinogenic snuff, nu-nu, *blown into his nose (right).*

methods, including massage, embrocations and sweating, to treat a wide range of diseases including those caused by infractions of the Mbyá moral code, environmental factors, parasites and microbial organisms. Like many indigenous peoples in Latin America, the Mbyá believe in the hot–cold classification of diseases. For eye ailments attributed to the cold, the Mbya wash the face and head with infusions of aromatic hot plants; with eye ailments attributed to the heat, cold running water and cold plants, such as the "tapir herb", are used.

Severe, inexplicable, mysterious illnesses that are resistant to regular diagnosis and therapeutic treatment are considered manifestations of evil (*pochy*) and are only amenable to spiritual methods of healing. Individuals who, out of laziness or choice, ignore the Mbyá spiritual practices of charity, love of fellow beings, the recital of sacred hymns and ritual dances become dominated by evil. Choosing to learn a "noxious science", they become sorcerers and inflict mysterious diseases or even death on their neighbours. There are also a number of illness-producing

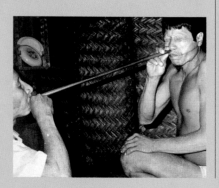

PLANT SPIRITS

As living entities, all plants and trees are inhabited by one or more spirits. Considered as the guardians and owners of an entire species of plants, the spirits' sphere of activity is global and immortal. Referred to as the mothers of the plants, these spirits may take a human or bird form.

The mother plant spirits are generally neither good nor bad in nature, although some are considered evil. The mightiest tree spirit, that of the lupuna tree (*Ceiba pentandra*) takes the form of a malign demon and sorcerer smoking a huge pipe. A group of plants known as piripiri, mostly belonging to the sedge genus *Cyperus*, have a sparrow-hawk as their master or owner. Some piripiri plant spirits are said to injure and sicken humans but most are used in childbirth, for open wounds, eye infections and hunting and love magic.

The mothers of the lupuna tree are associated with insanity, and tobacco mothers with migraine headaches. After determining which plant is causing a sickness, native curers heal the malignancy with the same plant. The mother spirit, as the inner, immaterial quality of each plant, is able to cure different diseases, so that healing is not merely the physical result of taking a preparation.

The mother spirits imbibe teas made of the same substance as their plant. They also like certain foods

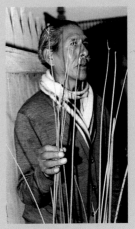

A Peruvian doctor with piripiri plants.

such as tobacco, and are attracted or charmed by the odour of piripiri and the seeds of the annatto tree.

---

evil spirits, including the unruly soul of the lapacho (*Tecoma obtusata*). This spirit manifests its malignancy by shooting injurious pebbles and leaves into human bodies. For this reason, the wood of the lapacho is never used in construction or for any other purpose.

The Aymara- and Quechua-speaking peoples of the Andes are the largest indigenous group in the Americas. They are primarily herders and farmers, living at altitudes of 8,800–14,000ft (2,700–4,300m). The most skilful Andean herbalists are the Kallawaya, who live in the high plateaus of mid-western Bolivia. Known as the Lords of the Medicine Bag for the woven saddle-bags in which they carry their herbs, Kallawaya herbalists are renowned throughout South America, and at the turn of the 19th century, people travelled from as far afield as Europe to be treated of supposedly incurable diseases by the Kallawaya.

Many Kallawaya herbalists have now set up clinics in urban centres to treat the stress-related diseases of rural migrants to the cities, but Kallawaya herbalists still constitute over 25 percent of the population in some thirty rural communities and are often the leaders in their villages. They collect their plants everywhere from alpine mountains to lowland tropical forests, yielding a rich inventory of herbs. They know of some 800 plants, of which 300 are used medicinally. In order to regulate dosage, control side effects and help families deal with an illness, Kallawaya herbalists stay in a patient's home during the treatment. A consequence of Kallawaya home therapy is the subsequent exchange of goods and services between the curer and family.

Kallawaya medicine is an open, dynamic system and a number of practitioners have introduced synthetic drugs and other medicines into their practice. Various Kallawaya herbalists specialize in diseases of different body organs, such as the kidney, liver and lungs. Kallawaya medicine is transmitted from father to son or through a male's apprenticeship to an expert herbalist, which may last 8 years.

Kallawaya curers maintain a spiritual relationship to Mother Earth, whose fluids issue to form, in various combi-

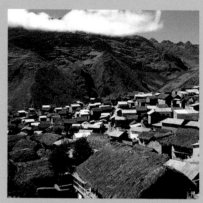

A Kallawaya village in the Bolivian mountains.

nations, the different plant species. In the form of plant-derived teas and other preparations, the fluids of Mother Earth are conveyed to human bodies.

CANDOMBLÉ

In the cities of northern Brazil a religious cult that practises possession by spirits dominates the lives of the urban poor. Termed Candomblé or Batuque, this religion is a synthesis of African, Catholic and Amazonian Indian ritual.

In Candomblé, plants play an important role in the fumigations, ritual baths and offerings prepared for the deities. All plants as well as parts of the human body correspond to specific deities. Plants belonging to a deity are used to cure diseases in that part of the body over which the deity holds sway.

In order to be effective at all, plants must be gathered according to certain prescribed rules. Anyone

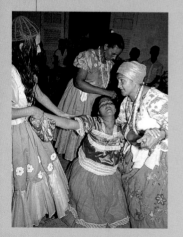

Candomblé dancers under the control of the spirits.

gathering wild plants should be wearing light-coloured clothing and be spiritually clean. Before picking the plant, permission must be requested by singing an incantation to the relevant deity and depositing a small offering. With certain plants, the sex of the person, the direction in which the plant grows and whether the left or right hand is used can be of great consequence. Plants are collected at specific times. The moon must be in a certain phase, or the sun at a particular position on a day dedicated to a certain deity. Since the various deities govern their own periods of the day the plants also change their qualities at different times of day.

Kallawaya medicine focuses on the dynamic and functional relationships of the individual organism with the macrocosmic environment. The tripartite division of the human body into head, trunk and legs is metaphorically and empirically linked to community topography, and the sections and parts of the mountains. Neglecting or maltreating the flocks and land, disturbing ancestral mountain sites and failing to maintain the mountain shrines creates disturbances in body–environment relationships, resulting in illness. Health is restored by depositing complex food offerings at mountain shrines that correspond to parts of the body.

Herbal therapy focuses on the interactions between organ systems, rather than on individual organs. Circulatory, digestive, reproductive and respiratory processes take place at the *sonoco* (comprising the heart–mind and gastrointestinal systems), which generates body fluids and excretory by-products. The decomposition and flow of nutrients to and from the *sonoco* is continuous and cyclical, and is thought to be produced by a hydraulic action that can also be seen in ritual behaviour, geological activity and plant physiology. Illness is diagnosed as resulting from the loss of vital fluids, or from dietary and environmental factors. Disturbances in blood circulation, the cyclical flow of body fluids and the excretion of waste products result in the accumulation of toxic substances. Diagnosis involves observing the colour and texture of the urine, the body temperature and the pulse, which all indicate that the blood may be too fast, slow, thick or thin. These readings are expressed as the blood being hot, cold, wet or dry. In general, slow and thick blood is indicative of arthritis, slow and thin blood of respiratory ailments, and fast and thin blood is symptomatic of tachycardia.

Medicinal plants are classified as being hot, warm, cordial or cold. Hot and warm plants speed up the flow of body fluids. Although most Kallawaya medicinal plants are native to South America, 18 plants, including borage, chamomile, fennel and garlic are of European origin.

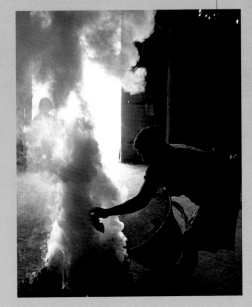

Coca leaves, a ubiquitous remedy in Kallawaya households, are used to treat gastrointestinal ailments, bruises, colds and other discomforts resulting from exposure to the high-altitude environment. In much of South America they are also valued for their stimulant properties. Here a Colombian Macuna woman burns coca leaves to release mood-altering alkaloids.

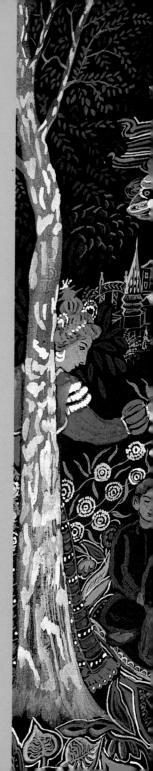

Plants and Visions

Plants that can evoke a profoundly religious experience when ingested have been termed entheogens: "that which gives rise to the god within us". In non-industrial societies, the ability of these plants to transcend the normal human sphere and to draw the taker into communication with different realms of existence has placed them within a complex web of mythical allusions and religious associations. In industrial societies, too, entheogens have been the subject of curiosity, wonder, controversy, fear and legislation.

Whether these plants are insidiously evil producers of private, hellish experiences or routes to a higher world depends on the reality in the mind of the beholder. The highly varied effects that entheogens trigger result from an interaction of the user's personality, emotional state, cultural background, motivations, expectations and the interpersonal and physical environment in which the experience takes place. In non-industrial societies these powerful plants are treated with profound respect. They are taken within a carefully codified religious context, with specific intentions – such as diagnosing disease – and after days of ritual purification. This culturally channelled procedure contrasts with the undisciplined, desacralized and recreational attitude of those people and societies that flirt with, or condemn and castigate, the use of such plants.

A hallucinogen-inspired painting of a sacred ceremony, by a member of a group of Peruvian shamans who are so skilled in the use of plants that they are known as vegetalistas.

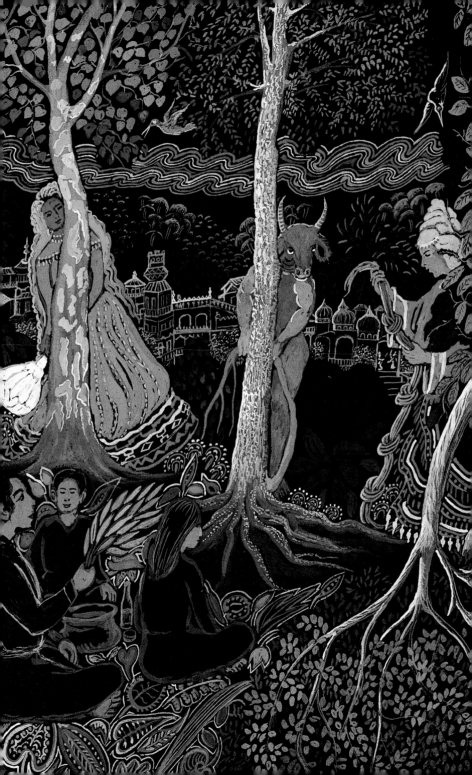

Peyote

Peyote (*Lophophora williamsii*) is a small, succulent, blue-green, spineless cactus, indigenous to the Chihuahuan Desert of northeastern Mexico and the Rio Grande Basin. The plant contains mescaline and forty-three other alkaloids with psychoactive, stimulant and medicinal properties. A similar psychoactive cactus, *Ariocarpus retusus*, is known as the "false peyote".

The Huichol Indians of the Sierra Madre Mountains of north-central Mexico have placed the peyote at the centre of their religious rituals and their cultural symbolism. According to Huichol tradition, peyote and maize both sprang from the body of an ancestral deity, Brother Deer. Maize, deer and peyote are, for the Huichol, of the same essence, and by ingesting peyote the Huichol assimilate the heart and

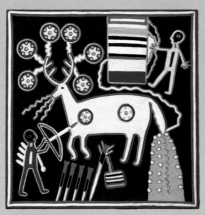

The Huichol are famous for their colourful yarn paintings, which often illustrate aspects of the peyote ritual. This yarn painting shows the magical transformation of the deer into a peyote as it is shot by the hunters at the culmination of the ancestors' first peyote hunt.

soul of the Deer-Person, and acquire his wisdom. Peyote is food for the soul, as maize and deer are nourishment for the body and, as manifestations of each other, it is necessary first to eat peyote and kill deer in order to plant maize.

In order to secure peyote for curing and for dry-season ceremonies, small groups of richly costumed pilgrims are dispatched by Huichol temples on a 300-mile (500-km), 6-week long visionary journey to Wirikúta, a sacred desert in the state of San Luis Potosi. In preparation for the journey, the pilgrims perform a ritual of confession and purification and during the journey both they and their relatives who remain behind forego sexual relations, washing and bathing, and also greatly minimize their food and water intake, excretion and sleep. In this manner, the pilgrims strive to discard their human condition and take on a divine, luminous presence.

The peyote pilgrimage, carried out in the late autumn to secure rain, abundant crops, health and children, is a return to the Huichol sacred land of origins and creation, the abode of the gods, ancestral shades and unborn children. With the shaman-leader representing Grandfather Fire and the pilgrims taking on the personae of other Huichol deities, the journey is a commemoration and and also a dramatized re-enactment of the exodus of the ancestral deities out of Wirikúta. The divine pilgrims stop and leave votive offerings and prayers at all sacred sites immortalized in the primordial peyote hunt of the ancestral deities.

The first peyote are collected on arrival at Wirikúta, and that evening

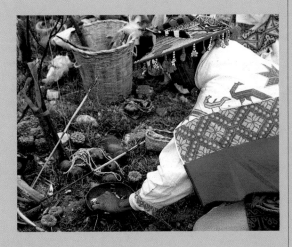

When the Huichol arrive at the sacred desert of Wirikúta after their long visionary journey, the first peyote plants to appear to the leading four pilgrim/deities as deer are shot with arrows from four directions. They are given rich offerings, reverently divided and then ritually distributed among the participants in the hunt. Here, a Huichol shaman divides the first peyote to be caught on the pilgrimage. The arrows that were used by the leading shaman to shoot the first cactus that he saw are visible on the left.

the pilgrims partake of their harvest, while they sing and dance around a fire. Huichol peyote experiences, being personal encounters with the deities, are private and incommunicable, but typically include messages and shamanic songs given by the deities appearing in animal form. On the return trip, flesh-and-blood deer are hunted by the pilgrims, and sacrificed in the cornfields to ensure fecundity and rain. By bringing them out of a sacred, untouchable condition, this homeward-bound ceremonial deer hunt also absolves the pilgrims from the strict privations of the journey. In a final, parched-maize ceremony,

ANCIENT WORSHIP

Known as the Flowers of the Divine Mother, peyote was used in pre-Colombian Mexico to treat fever, arthritis and other illnesses, to stimulate warriors in battle, overcome fatigue and to endure hunger and thirst. Peyote also served to communicate with the gods and to acquire knowledge of things to come.

After the Spanish Conquest, the use of peyote spread among the non-Indian population for the purpose of detecting thefts, divination

and fortune telling. In 1620, an edict was issued by the Inquisition forbidding, under the severest penalties, the use of peyote. The officials of the Inquisition, however, denied that peyote's remarkable effects were actually caused by the cactus. Instead, they were considered to be the work of Satan. However, the Inquisition was unsuccessful in stopping the use of peyote.

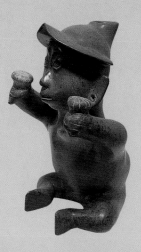

A mesoamerican tomb figurine of a hunchbacked dwarf holding a pair of peyote plants, c.200BC.

large amounts of peyote are consumed, while the pilgrims give a detailed account of their journey and sing all night about Father Sun, Brother Deer and the other gods.

Peyote is utilized as a sacrament by a religious movement known as the North American Church, whose members, consisting of 250,000 Native Americans, are distributed from the US Mexican border up to Alaska. Peyote ceremonies are held in times of trouble, to bring rain, for the well-being of humanity and, most frequently, for healing the sick. Preparation for the nocturnal ceremony consists of contemplation and fasting, sexual continence, rubbing with scented plants and, at times, taking a sweat bath.

The ceremony commonly takes place in a *tipi*, with the participants sitting

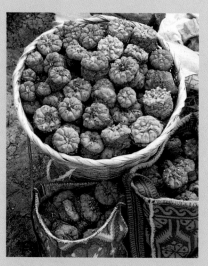

A basket and woven wool bags filled with peyote, from a Wirikúta pilgrimage. Some peyote-gourds can themselves represent deities.

cross-legged in a circle. At the centre is a crescent-shaped earthen altar which represents the moon, sacred mountains and Mother Earth, and ritual paraphernalia symbolizing many other spirit forces. A large peyote plant, Father Peyote, situated at the crest of the altar, and to which all prayers are directed, represents the Great Spirit. A groove traced from Father Peyote along the crescent marks the path of the worshippers' thoughts to the Great Spirit and the road of life and death that believers travel to gain knowledge of Peyote. The line also shows the trail of the plant's discoverer, Peyote Woman. Below the altar is a ceremonial fire, believed to be a curative spirit-force and represents the sun, life and heart.

After the group prays and smokes together, the dried peyote buttons are purified in cedar incense and pressed to the heart before being eaten. Shaking a gourd rattle, the leader or Roadman then sings the opening song, after which a staff, a drum and the rattle are passed around in a circle for each participant to sing four religious songs. The changing rhythms, triumphant or plaintive songs, blazing fire and fragrant smoke reinforce each other and elevate the intense, emotional prayers of the participants, as they quietly contemplate the fire and Father Peyote.

At midnight, when the participants' experiences are at their height, the fire-tender goes outside to blow four times on an eagle-bone whistle, imitating the shrill cries of an approaching eagle. This announces that at midnight all things – day and night, man and woman, the six directions – are unified in the middle of the *tipi*. The Roadman

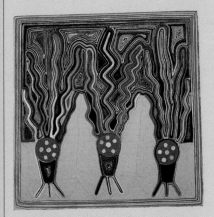

A Huichol yarn painting of a peyote must show the entire cactus, down to its roots. Ritual peyote use diffused to the Tonkawa and Lipan Apache of the Texas Gulf in the early 19th century. It was taken up by the Plains peoples in the 1890s.

sings the Midnight Song four times, after which water is distributed to the participants. At this point, prayers are recited or a curing ritual performed for the sick. The singing, drumming and rattling continue until morning and increase in power as the effect of the peyote deepens. At daybreak, the Roadman's wife, representing Dawn or Peyote Woman, brings in a ceremonial breakfast, consisting of water, parched corn, dried, sweet meat and fruit. The meeting is concluded by the Roadman singing to the morning star. The group then rests, talks and composes new songs suggested by the night's experience. At noon, a feast is served at which a single spoon must be used by the entire company.

MEDIUM AND MESSAGE

The peyote religion regards the plant as an incarnation of a divine being and messenger, enabling communion with the Great Spirit without the medium of a priest. Peyote is used as a medicine for the soul and for illnesses such as tuberculosis, pneumonia, influenza and scarlet fever. Each individual learns church doctrines through intense, sacred encounters with the plant and is free to interpret them as he or she wishes. Devotees partake of the plant with sincerity, concerted effort and in the state of ritual purity needed to commune with the Great Spirit. This provides a powerful religious experience in which the solutions to numerous personal problems are obtained.

Merely taking peyote is, however, not sufficient. In "taking the Peyote Road" members must lead a life of humility and altruistic love, look upon evil with pity, injustice with compassion and misfortune with indifference. Most do not experience visions, which should not be sought other than to reveal moral transgressions and impurities of the soul.

During a North American Church ceremony, the fire-tender shapes the ashes from the ceremonial fire into a water or thunder bird, the messenger of peyote, which represents the source of all life and the revelations of peyote to the devotee.

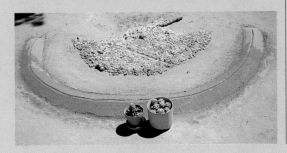

Sacred mushrooms

Several different species of psilocybe mushrooms, as well as a number of other entheogenic plants, are used by the Chatino, Mixtec, Mixe and other native peoples of southern Mexico. These mushrooms contain two hallucinogenic alkaloids, psilocyn and psilocybin, which act by inhibiting the nerve-impulse transmitter, serotonin. (A beta-blocker, sold under the trade name "Visken" and used to treat high blood pressure and regulate cardiac function, has been developed from psilocybin.) The sacred mushrooms are primarily taken by mesoamerican peoples in cases of intractable illness, but also to learn the whereabouts of any lost or stolen articles, or to resolve problems and conflicts. The medicinal and divinatory efficacy of the mushrooms is believed to be a result of their mythical emergence from the blood of Christ or the bones of ancient sages and prophet-kings.

Taking the mushrooms can cause adverse reactions, or even death, if the prescribed preparations – refraining from sexual contact, certain foods, agricultural labour, expressing anger and injuring the earth's living creatures – are not adhered to. The solemn period of 4 or more days of preparation are devoted to praying before the family altar or in church for forgiveness and permission to take the sacred mushrooms. The mushrooms are gathered by a young virgin, or a prayer is recited before they are picked. They are always handled with great care and reverence, and are placed on the house altar or in church.

On the morning of a propitious day, a bath and simple breakfast are taken, but nothing is eaten after noon. The plants are ingested at night in an isolated house, free from the disturbances and noise which cause the mushrooms to stop "speaking". A shaman may take the mushrooms on behalf

A mushroom effigy sculpture from highland Guatemala, c.500 BC.

DIVINATION

One of the most widespread hallucinogenic mushrooms is the fly agaric. It was used by the Koryak and other Siberian peoples to divine the future, diagnose illnesses and dreams and to learn the condition of dead relatives in the celestial realm. There are reports of the ritual use of fly agaric along the northwest Pacific coast, by the Dogrib of northwestern Canada and the Ojibway of the Great Lakes.

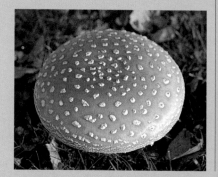

The fly agaric mushroom, Amanita muscaria.

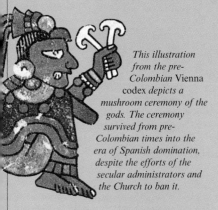

This illustration from the pre-Colombian Vienna codex *depicts a mushroom ceremony of the gods. The ceremony survived from pre-Colombian times into the era of Spanish domination, despite the efforts of the secular administrators and the Church to ban it.*

that was said. Once the drug has taken effect, the individual initiates a dialogue with a visionary boy and girl, diminutive elderly people, saints, a deceased relative or some other spirit personage. Sometimes there are no apparitions, only a voice, which asks why the sacred plants were taken. The imbiber explains the reason and, in the case of illness, if there is a visionary figure it proceeds to heal with massage, sucking and other indigenous therapeutic methods. Alternatively, the spirit of the plant announces the cause of the illness and advises on the ritual means that can be used to alleviate it. To an observer, the person who has taken the mushrooms appears to be conducting an extended, two-way conversation, with a different voice according to whether the patient or the spirit of the plant is speaking.

of a client, at times combining this with divination by means of maize kernels or complex parcels of eggs, feathers, bark and other materials. Alternatively, the person with a problem may imbibe the mushrooms personally, attended by one or two relatives or trusted friends who monitor the proceedings so that the individual can later be informed of all

SPIRIT VOICES

Among the Mazatecs, the extended family of a sick person takes part in a nocturnal vigil presided over by a shaman. Sacred mushrooms are blessed and ingested by the whole group and, out of darkness and silence, the shaman begins to speak on behalf of the sick person, singing, chanting and praying with increasing intensity. The spirits of the mushrooms speak through the shaman and evoke the shaman's inspired capacity to utter divine words of power in a poetic, mournful and ecstatic manner, leading to a spiritual and therapeutic catharsis. The group responds

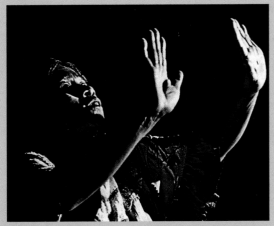

Maria Sabina, a Mazatec shaman, enters a trance.

to the canticles and prayers of the shaman, invoking God, the saints and forces of nature. In the spiritual songs, the mushroom spirits heal via the divine word or Logos.

Datura

The use of datura in coming-of-age rites of passage was common among Californian and Algonkian-speaking Native Americans. The neophytes experienced dreams and visions in which they acquired animal guardian spirits, learned special songs and, in the case of the Delaware, were informed of their

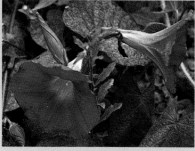

In South America, daturas such as these take the form of small trees with huge, colourful, trumpet-shaped flowers. Widely cultivated as ornamental plants in house-yards and gardens, these Brugmansia *species are chemically similar to herbaceous daturas and are employed from Colombia to Chile to commune with the spirit world, to find lost objects and treasure, foresee the future, and to treat asthma, bronchitis, tumours, swollen infections and joints, muscle cramps, and other ailments. Smelling the fragrant flowers is said to cause headaches, but in southern Colombia people with insomnia walk through* Brugmansia-*lined streets in the evening to induce sleep. The Shuar of Ecuador, among others, administer tree datura infusions to unruly children for the ancestors to visit and admonish them, and even feed datura to their dogs to make them locate more game. At puberty, Shuar youths drink a tree datura infusion in order to become brave warriors, eligible for marriage. Tree datura intoxication produces an initial state of confusion followed by an extended period of sleep, accompanied by a series of coloured dream visions which continue sporadically for 1–4 days.*

past lives and future occupations. Zuni priests used datura as an anaesthetic in setting fractured bones and performing surgery, as well as administering it to clients for contacting ancestral spirits and ascertaining the identity of thieves.

The mind-altering and medicinal properties of datura have long been known to the Arabs, Persians and Hindus. Because datura contains the highly toxic alkaloids scopolamine and hyoscyamine, ingestion can result in amnesia, disorientation, burning thirst, temporary blindness, paralysis, coma and death. Datura has been used by criminals in India, Tanzania, Peru and other parts of the world to stupefy and murder their victims. The Chibcha of Colombia administered it to wives and slaves before burying them alive with deceased chiefs and warriors. Datura is also said to be an aphrodisiac and has been used as a beer additive in Europe, China and Peru.

The Kamsá and Inga of the Sibundoy Valley in Colombia maintain a great diversity of tree datura (*Brugmansia*) types. As cultivars, tree daturas do not occur in the wild and cannot reproduce sexually or by self-propagation. By means of stem cuttings, the Sibundoy have selected and reproduced twelve clones, varieties, and hybrids which are genetically distinct and breed true to type. Each of these cultivars is the hereditary property of particular families, who use them for different medicinal and psychoactive purposes. One cultivar, for example, is used to treat rheumatic limbs and joints, another as a vermifuge (dewormer) and three less toxic cultivars are employed as psychoactive drugs by shamans.

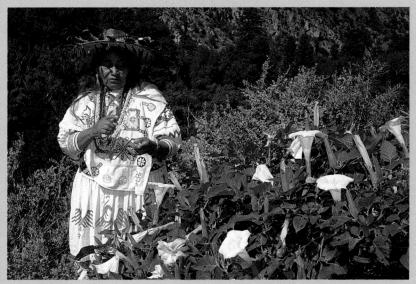

A Mexican Huichol woman offers a prayer against datura, which is considered to be a great sorcerer.

PUBERTY RITES

Datura (or *mondzo*) is used by the Shangana-Tsonga of northern Transvaal and Mozambique to exorcise alien spirits, as an ordeal poison to disclose sorcerers and criminals, and in the girls' nubility ritual, which is carried out to ensure fecundity and provide eligibility for marriage.

Tsonga marriages are contracted by means of bridewealth payments (in which the groom pays for his future wife) and barrenness would result in disgrace and financial disaster for the family. Upon reaching nubility, Tsonga girls are secluded in a hut, taught women's roles and undergo various privations and rituals, involving purificatory immersion in water, lacerations, labia minora elongation, and defloration with a kudu horn. On the last day of 3 months of ritual, the girls ingest *mondzo* or "that which opens one's eyes". Wearing blue dresses and face paint, the novices first execute a series of mimes and energetic dances representing stages from infancy to sexual maturity, which end when the officiant or "school mother" sprays saliva over the novices, symbolizing the crossing over water to adulthood. She then places straw-encrusted clay cubes between the legs of the initiates to signify the regrowth of the pubic hair which, as an act of separation, had been shaved previously. The initiates are administered small doses of datura tea, and in their "journey of fantasy" they hear the voices of the ancestor-gods and see bluish-green patterns, which represent the gods in the form of small snakes. (Drumming rhythms produce visual patterns during the dancing and intensify the effects of the plant drug.) The novices are neither sickened nor poisoned by the datura. Finally they are given new names and clothes for their reincorporation into Tsonga society as mature women.

Health and Beauty

There is a growing interest in cultivating, collecting, preparing and using herbs, not only in cookery but also in the preparation of home remedies and even cosmetics. Plants have been used for thousands of years to embellish and entice and, until recently, were the main constituents of cosmetics and perfumes. Many fruits, vegetables and herbs possess oils and vitamins which nourish and improve the condition of the skin. The delicately scented perfumes of flowers and plants produce a feeling of relaxation and comfort and their heady volatile oils have an uplifting and stimulating effect upon the emotions and nerves.

Commercial soaps and hair colourants contain alkalis which neutralize the acidic, antibacterial coating of the skin. Store-bought cosmetics contain mineral oils which deprive the skin of fat-soluble vitamins, and antioxidants and other additives which ensure a long shelf-life but are readily absorbed by the skin, with unknown, long-term effects. Herbal preparations are economical and satisfying ways to natural beauty and health, and are most beneficial when freshly applied, because the effective vitamins and minerals will have had no occasion to decompose or evaporate.

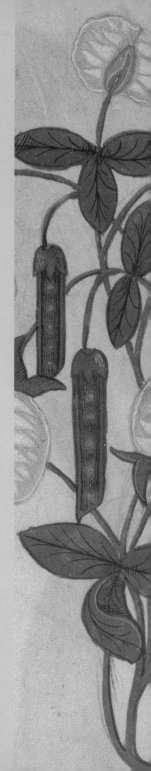

The rose, one of the oldest sources of perfumes, and the pea, one of the oldest cultivated foods (examples having been found fossilized in Swiss lake villages), shown side by side in a 16th-century English herbal.

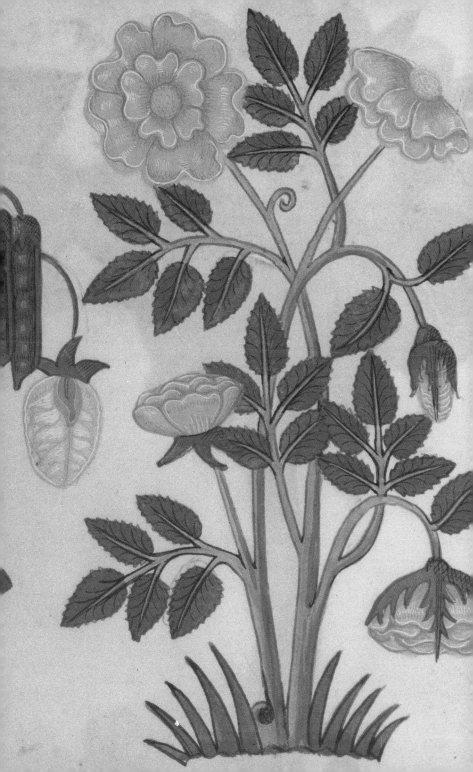

The cultivation of herbs

The common garden herbs are tolerant of soil conditions, although results will be better if they are grown in their preferred soil types. Wormwood, rosemary, lady's mantle, chicory, hyssop, lavender, horehound, mint, marjoram, oregano, sage, thyme and juniper prefer alkaline soil. Lemon balm, lavender, borage, centaury, Roman chamomile, coriander, fennel and thyme like sandy

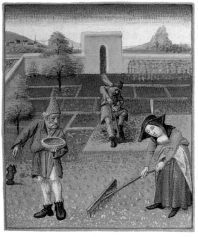

Books on garden design and plant-tending, such as De Rustican, *which contains this illustration of seed-sowing, first became popular in Europe in the 15th century.*

soils. Most other herbs prefer a friable loam that is neutral or slightly alkaline. If the soil is acidic, a sprinkling of limestone or ashes will help plants take up nutrients. Hyssop and lemon balm prefer poor soils, and Mediterranean herbs produce more oils if the soil is not too rich. Herbs prefer well-drained soil. If the soil drains poorly, add peat moss, leaf mould, wood chips or compost.

Annuals and most biennials are planted outdoors in mid-to-late spring after the soil has warmed up, and the danger of frost is over. Carefully remove weeds but do not transplant them by depositing them in the compost heap. Turn soil to a depth of 1ft (30cm), breaking up the clods to create a fine tilth. Allow the soil to settle for at least a week before planting any seed, and if the soil feels heavy and lumpy, spread a fine layer of sand along the seed-furrow. Cover the seeds with a thin sprinkling of soil, firm in with a smooth board and moisten the seedbed with a fine spray. To deter seed-eating birds, cover the bed with a mesh screening until the seeds have germinated.

Apply a dressing of manure or compost every summer. Before a heavy frost, perennials should be dug up, put into pots and stored indoors. Bring the plants indoors in intermediate stages by placing them in a cool garage for a few nights to ease the transition. For added protection during the winter, cover the roots of mature shrubs with compost. Mullein, columbines, elder bushes, gladioli, lavender, marigolds and primrose all protect the herb bed from the wind. To rid the herbs of plant lice, spray the affected plants with an infusion of 2lb (1kg) of stinging nettles steeped in water for several hours.

Plants that are slow to germinate, such as parsley, and rare or unfamiliar seeds, as well as basil, sage, marjoram and thyme, are best started indoors in late winter or early spring, and transplanted to the garden when the ground is warm. As a germination medium, use a loamless seed-growing mixture or equal parts of coarse sand, peat or

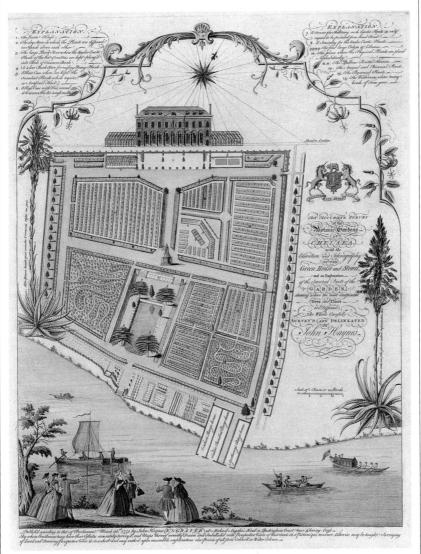

An engraving by John Haynes, from 1751, showing the plan of the Chelsea Physic Garden in London. Large-scale botanical gardens had begun to be built throughout Britain, France, Germany, Holland and Italy in the 16th and 17th centuries. They were often attached to universities and medical schools to provide the raw materials for both botanical and medical scholarship.

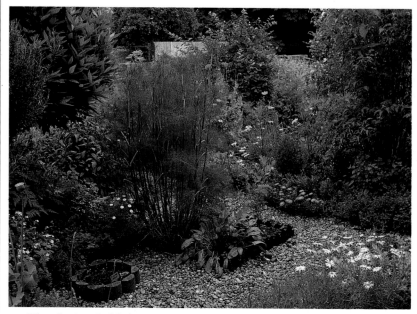

When planning a herb bed, it is wise to plant herbs that require different amounts of water at different ends of the bed. Plant herbs that need less sun near taller plants and plant aggressive herbs, such as lemon balm and mints, separately or contain the roots with divider boards.

sphagnum moss, sterilized garden loam and fertilizer, blended and passed through a mesh sieve. Firm the mixture down into the container and place the seeds into shallow furrows 2in (5cm) apart. Sprinkle over a fine layer of potting mixture, to a depth of twice the seed's diameter. Fine seeds should be pressed into the soil. Firm the soil down and water well with a fine spray. Cover the soil surface with a wet newspaper and glass plate and place the pot in a warm spot, around 20°C (70°F) and away from direct sunlight.

Seeds need to be misted several times a day until they germinate, at which point remove the covering and expose them to good light but not direct sunlight. When the second pair of leaves forms, transplant the seedlings to a larger pot with a slightly richer soil. Handle seedlings by the leaves to avoid damaging the tiny new roots and stems, and keep the plants out of direct sunlight for a day or two until they recover from the shock of planting. Move the plants outside gradually by placing them in a sheltered, shady location and taking them in at night for several days.

Most of the smaller culinary herbs that are grown indoors thrive in a temperature of 16–20°C (60–70°F), with parsley, rosemary and burnet preferring a cooler temperature of 16°C (60°F).

Many herbs require 6–8 hours of sunlight a day, but mints and parsley prefer partial shade for most of the day, with 1–2 hours of sun in the morning or late afternoon. Do not place plants in direct draughts, in front of or above heat outlets or air conditioners. Kitchens may be too hot and dry, with cooking fumes and large temperature variations. When planting several herbs in one container, use only those that require similar watering, sun and soil conditions. Mint, parsley and lemon verbena are planted separately, because they overcrowd other plants.

Check soil moisture every other day and each day in hot weather. Seedlings need daily watering. For added humidity, set a container of water next to the plants and a layer of sphagnum moss on the soil's surface. Culinary herbs that are regularly harvested need a weak liquid fertilizer every 2 weeks from spring to autumn, but not during the winter. Occasionally, set the pots in a kitchen sink or bathtub and flush excess salts by watering and rewatering for a half hour or so. Perennials, particularly mint, fill the pots with roots and need repotting every year or two.

OTHER METHODS OF PROPAGATION

A hardy, non-woody perennial can be dug up in early spring and divided for replanting. Pull it apart or use a knife to divide the plant into smaller sections, taking care not to damage the roots. Each root should have an attached shoot or stem. Replant and water thoroughly. Nurture until the roots have established themselves. Certain plants, such as French tarragon, are divided in autumn.

In the late summer, take 3–6in (8–15cm) stem cuttings of non-flowering, perennial plants from just above the semi-hardwood, by making a clean cut at a 45° angle. Remove the leaves from the lower third of a cutting, dip it in water and insert it into a pot containing a mix of equal parts milled sphagnum and perlite, or two parts sand and one part vermiculite. Cover the pot with a plastic bag so as not to touch the leaves, but aerate the plant every few days. Spray the leaves lightly and frequently during dry weather. Cuttings are transplanted to potting soil when they have acquired roots about 1in (3cm) long. When the cuttings show signs of growth, place them in a sunny, sheltered place and add fertilizer.

To make root cuttings, dig up tender plants that have long taproots in the spring or late autumn. Carefully cut the root into short pieces – some 2–3in (5–8cm) long – and insert root pieces which have a bud, from which new shoots and roots can grow, just below the surface of the potting soil.

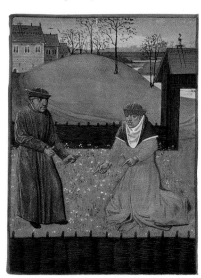

An anonymous 15th-century painting of a rustic being taught how to tend a herb garden.

Collection and drying

Medicinal herbs should generally be collected at the beginning of the blossoming period in clear, dry, weather, in the early morning after the dew has evaporated. Plants with volatile oils, such as the mints and lemon balm, are gathered just before noon. Mint, hyssop, lavender, rosemary and thyme are collected when the flowers are fullest, and sage when the buds first appear.

Flowers are gathered immediately upon opening, before they are fully expanded. Leaves are collected in the spring, when they are young but developed and the flowers are in bud. Stems are collected when the flowers are beginning to open. Fruits are gathered when they are ripe and the stalks are dry. Bulbs should be collected when the leaves of the plant are falling off. Roots are best gathered in the evening, before the plant begins to form flowers or in the autumn. Bark is harvested in the early spring or in the autumn.

The identity of the plants collected should be checked carefully. Several medicinal plants in the carrot family (*Umbelliferae*), for example, are similar to their poisonous relatives. It is a good idea not to collect near highways, heavily used roads, industrial plants or in areas that are sprayed with pesticides.

Medicinal herbs should be dried quickly and carefully in a warm, dark part of the home with a good current of air to prevent fermentation. Herbs are best dried when spread in single, thin layers on elevated wire screen trays for 3–7 days. To dry seeds, the whole plant is dried for 5–6 days, the stems and pods then removed and the seeds left on the rack for another 7–10 days, and turned frequently. In cool or humid weather, a heater will maintain a steady

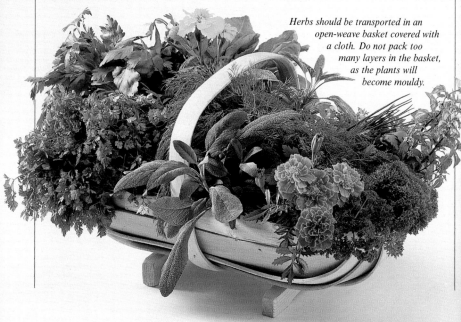

Herbs should be transported in an open-weave basket covered with a cloth. Do not pack too many layers in the basket, as the plants will become mouldy.

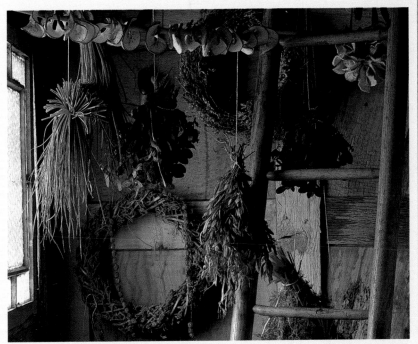

Herbs such as sage, thyme and sweet marjoram may be tied into loose bunches and hung in a dry, airy room or attic for a week. If the room cannot be darkened, place paper bags, with the bottoms cut out, over the bunches. Tender, freshly picked culinary herbs, such as basil, chives, dill, parsley and fennel, are best frozen. They can be added to cooking food direct from the freezer, or defrosted for salads.

temperature, and drying may be completed by spreading the herbs on a baking sheet and placing them in an oven at 38°C (100°F) for a few minutes. Roots and bark are cut into pieces 1in (2.5 cm) thick and dried for 6 weeks, while being turned over twice weekly. When dry, the leaves should be brittle, flower petals should rustle and bark and roots should snap smartly. Artificial heat can also be used throughout the drying process, at a temperature of 32–39°C (89–102°F), but the herbs need to be checked regularly for scorching.

When thoroughly dried, the leaves are removed from stems, except for aromatic plants with a high content of volatile oils, which are best stored whole. Herbs should be kept in airtight containers, made of wood or coloured glass, in a dry, cool, dark place. During the first week, check for any moisture or condensation inside the container, which shows that the herbs are not completely dried. Also check the herbs once a month for mildew and insect infestation. Dried herbs generally become inactive after about 6 months.

Herbal preparations

Infusions are prepared by steeping leaves and flowers in water that is below boiling point to extract aromatic, volatile compounds, while decoctions are prepared by boiling roots, bark, seeds and other hard plant material to obtain bitter, resinous constituents. Different herbs may need different methods of preparation, and different preparations of the same herb may yield dissimilar chemical constituents. A hot infusion of boneset, for example, induces perspiration, but a cold infusion is taken as a mild laxative.

Dried leaves for infusions and teas can be ground using a pestle and mortar. Standard infusions are prepared with 1.5oz (50g) of dried herbs to 2 pints (1 litre) of distilled water, or 1–2 teaspoonfuls of herbs to 1 cup of water. Plant material should be moistened with a little cold water before pouring on any hot water. Flowers and bitter herbs are steeped for 3–5 minutes, tougher plant parts for 10–15 minutes. Keep the infusion covered while it is steeping. Then strain and express the juice. A more active preparation results from setting the plant material for 10 hours in cold water, then bringing it to the boil and steeping for 10 minutes. Certain herbs, such as bilberry, cinque-foil, oak bark and thyme, are best added to cold water, brought to a boil, cooked for 3–15 minutes and allowed to cool, but drunk while still warm. Bearberry, burdock root, mistletoe and centaury are set in cold water for 5–12 hours, strained and taken cold or warmed slightly. Herbs to treat asthma, bronchitis and other mucosal ailments should also be set in cold water for several hours, then slowly warmed.

The normal ratio for fresh leaves is 3 teaspoonfuls for each cup of water. Bruise the leaves first by crushing them in a clean cloth, and prepare them in the same way as dried leaves. Seeds should also be bruised slightly with a pestle and mortar before being added to boiling water and simmered gently for 5–10 minutes.

A 15th-century fresco from the Villa d'Isogna in Val d'Aosta, Italy, showing a pharmacy and contemporary methods of herbal preparation.

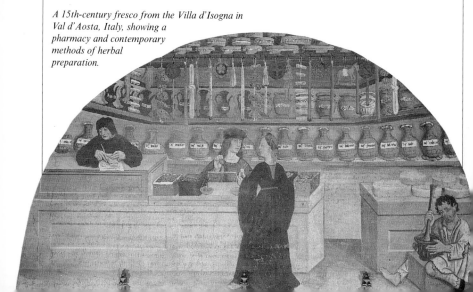

Decoctions require the same plant material/water ratio as infusions. Place the dried plant material in a medium-sized vessel with cold water and slowly bring to the boil. Reduce the heat and let the water simmer gently for 10–30 minutes, depending upon the hardness of the plant material, all the time keeping a lid on the vessel. Remove from the heat and let the decoction steep until cool. Pour it through a strainer, expressing the juices from the plant material. If the bark or root is used in combination with other plant parts, it should be cooked first, and the boiling decoction poured over the desired leaves or flowers and strained after 10–20 minutes.

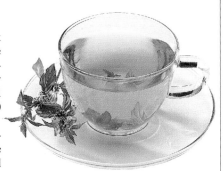

The flavour of aromatic herbs and flowers can be ruined if they are steeped for too long. If a stronger infusion is required, use more herbs. Medicinal teas are more active without sugar, but lemon and honey are ideal additives (honey promotes the loosening of mucus in throat and pectoral ailments). Those with fever should drink medicinal teas cold. They should be taken 2–3 times a day, slowly and in small sips.

Plant juices for internal and external use can be obtained with the aid of a juicing machine (the plant material should be covered with cold water for several minutes before placing it into the juicer). Alternatively, macerate the herbs and roots in a mortar or with a knife. After soaking them in water for half an hour, press the juice out using a fine cloth. A teaspoonful of juice can be taken straight or mixed with water, whey or milk.

To prepare a tincture, fill a screw-topped glass container with the herbs and add 70 percent (140 proof) alcohol. The tightly closed container must be kept in a warm place for 2 weeks and shaken twice a day before the liquid is strained. Fluid extracts may be prepared by adding herbs to a light, dry wine (1 part plant to 20 parts fluid). Soak for 10 days, away from direct sunlight and at a temperature of 15–20°C (59–68°F). Filter or squeeze through a clean cloth into a dark bottle, which should immediately be capped or corked. Drink no more than a small liquor glass of extract at one time.

Non-irritant plants can be placed directly on to an affected body part. Fresh herbs are first macerated, and dry herbs are moistened with hot water or herbal tea. Keep the poultice in place with a clean, warm cloth for no more than half an hour before applying a fresh one. Stronger-acting herbs are placed in small linen or muslin bags, dipped briefly in boiling water and cooled to 50°C (120°F) before being applied. Compresses are prepared by soaking linen or cotton in herbal infusions, tinctures or extracts. Hand towels may also be immersed in a hot herbal infusion, wrung out well and quickly applied. Keep the hot compress in place with a loose muslin bandage or dry towel. Prepare another compress after 3 minutes and keep alternating hot compresses for 10–30 minutes.

Foods that cure and preserve

The role of vitamins and other necessary food substances in dietary diseases such as scurvy, rickets, pellagra and beriberi is well known. Diets that are high in cholesterol and polyunsaturated fats have been widely reported as harming the cardiovascular system, and many authorities have noted the benefits of consuming less fat of all kinds, fewer animal foods and more plant-based oils. Diets that are high in animal protein and saturated fats and low in fresh vegetables and fibre are directly related to the occurrence of colon, prostate, breast and ovarian cancer.

Too high an intake of fat and, to a lesser extent, sugar and white flour products which are then converted to surplus energy and fat, also promotes the development of most cancers. Overeating in general causes an increase in the amounts of certain hormones and fatty acids which directly stimulate the growth of breast-cancer cells.

The milling and over-refinement of whole grains, which remove some 70 percent of the total protein, starch, minerals and vitamins have also been strongly linked to diabetes, heart disease, obesity and ulcers. In addition to

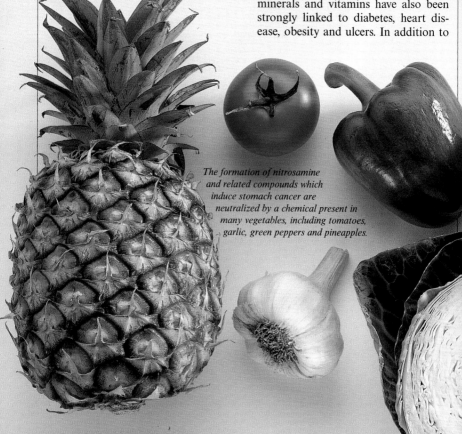

The formation of nitrosamine and related compounds which induce stomach cancer are neutralized by a chemical present in many vegetables, including tomatoes, garlic, green peppers and pineapples.

the well-known vitamins and fibre, food plants contain literally thousands of interacting biochemicals which have no nutritional value, but are nevertheless beneficial in slowing up or reversing the onset and progression of cancer.

Broccoli, cauliflower and other members of the cabbage family contain a chemical, indole-3-carbinol, which stimulates enzymes that cause the body to metabolize a harmless form of oestrogen, rather than the highly reactive form that is linked to breast cancer. Other chemicals that are present in the cabbage group and in hot peppers keep toxic molecules from binding to DNA, which may initiate cancer. Fibre in cereals, fruits and vegetables lowers blood cholesterol and impedes the growth of cancer-promoting enzymes in the delicate mucosal tissue of the colon. Even if cancerous growths have formed, genistein, a chemical found in soybeans and cabbage-family vegetables, deters the proliferation of cancerous cells and blocks the growth of new capillaries that are essential for certain tumours to develop and spread.

Garlic and related vegetables neutralize the ability of cancer-causing chemicals to transform normal cells into cancerous ones and may inhibit the early development of altered cells into full malignancy. Purslane, flaxseed and leafy vegetables contain linolenic acid which helps to build up the immune

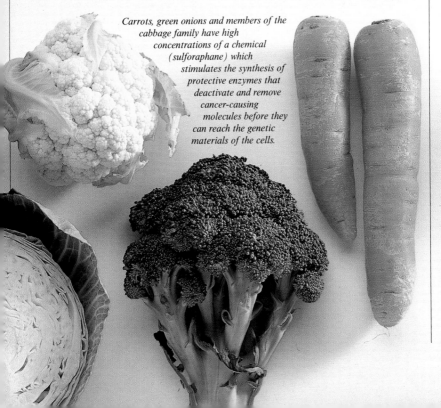

Carrots, green onions and members of the cabbage family have high concentrations of a chemical (sulforaphane) which stimulates the synthesis of protective enzymes that deactivate and remove cancer-causing molecules before they can reach the genetic materials of the cells.

system and deters heart disease.

The foods associated with a lower risk of cancers of all sorts are the green, leafy and cruciferous vegetables and yellow-orange fruits and vegetables. Dietary and nutritional factors may account for up to 35 percent of all cancers, and eating fruits and vegetables three times daily cuts the risk of certain cancers in half. Moderate exercise and a balanced and varied diet, low in calories and fats, with plenty of fruits, vegetables and fibre, is the best way to escape cancer and cardiovascular disease. Cancer-fighting plant chemicals are, happily, unchanged by food processing, and store-bought supplements are not as effective as the synergistic bioactivity of fresh food plants, processed at home (see pp.14–15).

The vitamins in plants not only maintain the health of the body but, by neutralizing the highly reactive and electrically charged molecules known as free oxygen radicals, are potentially active disease fighters as well. Free radicals are produced by air pollution, radiation, ozone, tobacco smoke, pesticides, dietary fats and by normal body metabolism. They are unstable and can damage critical cell molecules by adversely altering their chemistry. They can reprogramme genes, and have been implicated in more than 60 diseases, including cataracts, rheumatoid arthritis, heart disease and cancer. Because

Steaming is a far healthier method of cooking than boiling, as it preserves more nutrients. Pressure cooking also saves many nutrients. At the same time, baking is healthier than frying.

Diets that are rich in foods such as tomatoes, strawberries, aubergines or eggplants, beetroot or beets and turnips have been statistically linked to a lower than average risk of contracting many different forms of cancer.

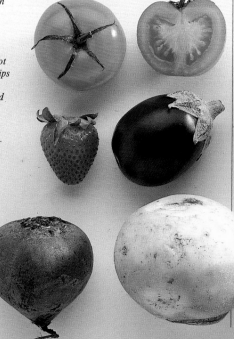

they have lost an electron, free radicals have a powerful tendency to bond to other molecules, including genetic material, resulting in an alteration of a cell's genetic code. They can also oxidize (rob an electron from) cholesterol, which helps it to adhere to artery walls, thereby contributing to heart disease. Most radicals are converted by the body's antioxidant enzymes into harmless compounds.

Vitamin C (found in citrus fruits, melons, tomatoes and green leafy vegetables), vitamin E (in wheat germ, oatmeal, nuts and brown rice) and beta carotene (in carrots, leafy green vegetables, citrus fruits and sweet potatoes) are powerful antioxidant compounds which counter free radical formation, sponge up harmful free radicals, prevent the oxidation of cells and the ensuing damage to DNA that can lead to cancer. Eating plant foods rich in these natural radical scavengers has protective value against heart disease, hardening of the arteries and cancer of the mouth, throat, stomach, pancreas, cervix, lung and breast. Since vitamin C and other vitamins are destroyed in cooking water, broccoli, potatoes and spinach should at most be lightly cooked in small amounts of water. The cooking water should not be thrown away but used in soups and gravies.

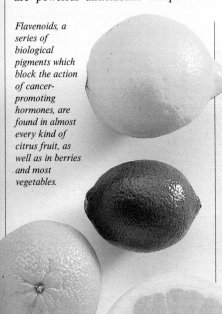

Flavenoids, a series of biological pigments which block the action of cancer-promoting hormones, are found in almost every kind of citrus fruit, as well as in berries and most vegetables.

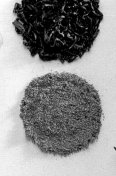

Rosemary (right), green tea (top) and the yellow pigment in curry (above) are all known to suppress cancer growth and reduce the activity of elements that induce cellular mutations.

Soups

CHINESE CHICKEN SOUP (SERVES 1)

1 chicken drumstick
1 thin slice of ginger
salt
2 spring onions or scallions

In Chinese medicine, chicken soup tonifies the blood and *ch'i* (see pp.82–5), and warms the stomach, spleen and liver. However, it can also take on a whole range of healing properties through the addition of the right herbal ingredients. To make the basic soup, take the flesh off the drumstick, and boil the bone in 2 cups of water with a little salt, the ginger and the spring onion, or scallion, whites. Simmer until the liquid is reduced to 1 cup, and skim. Bring back to a rapid boil and add the finely sliced chicken flesh with the spring onion, or scallion, greens. Cook for just 1–2 minutes, until the flesh turns white.

Add black wood ear mushrooms (*1*) to lower blood pressure and cholesterol. The same effect can be be achieved by adding a few Shiitake mushrooms (*2*). Add some Chinese box-thorn berries (*3, 9*) to cure excess liver yang, which reveals itself in headaches and sore, reddened eyes. High blood pressure can be tackled with Chinese or English celery (*4*). In Chinese medicine, the above are all thought to give the soup cooling properties. A mixture of Chinese red dates (*5*) and dang gui (*6*) can be added to make a bitter tonic for the old, the anaemic and for new mothers. A combination of shan yao (*7*), huang shi (*8*), box-thorn berries (*3, 9*) and dang shen (*10*) tonify *ch'i* and improve eyesight. To make warming soups, add walnuts (*11*) for the kidneys, or dried chestnuts (*12*) to remedy weakness in the lower back and knees.

ROSEHIP SOUP (SERVES 6)

2 ¹/₄ lb (1kg) ripened rosehips
12 ¹/₂ cups (3 litres) water
4 tablespoons (50g) cornflour
¹/₄ cup (25g) almonds
sugar
cream
sweet rusks

Rosehips have tonic effects, and help fight excess wind. Trim off the stalks and rinse. Simmer the rosehips for 3 hours, then strain and return to simmer. Add sugar to taste. Cream the cornflour with a little cold water and mix into the soup, stirring constantly. Cook for 5 minutes. Scald the almonds; remove the skins and chop. Add to soup. Serve with cream and sweet rusks.

LOVAGE SOUP (SERVES 4)

1 bunch of chopped fresh lovage leaves and stems
6 tablespoons (75g) butter
1 chopped garlic clove
1 handful of roughly chopped parsley
2 chopped sticks of celery
grated nutmeg
salt and pepper
2 small slices (50g) brown bread
2 ³/₄ pints (1 ¹/₂ litres) of meat or vegetable stock
¹/₄ pint (150ml) thick or double cream

Lovage is a diuretic and a stimulant, and also helps to relieve flatulence, but should not be overconsumed, as this can lead to kidney problems. Although the small quantities of lovage used in this recipe are harmless, in general the herb should be avoided by pregnant women. To prepare the soup, melt the butter in a pan and gently cook the garlic, parsley, celery and a pinch each of nutmeg, salt and pepper. After 2–3 minutes add the chopped lovage. Soak the bread in some of the stock for 2 minutes then squeeze it out and add it to the other ingredients in the pan, stirring well. Bring the stock to the boil, pour gradually over the other ingredients and simmer for 10 minutes. Liquidize or put through a coarse strainer. Return to the pan and reheat. Stir in the cream off the heat just before serving.

ELDERBERRY SOUP (SERVES 4)

Elder has been claimed to relieve pulmonary problems, purify the blood and induce perspiration. Wash the clusters and remove the stems. Add the cinnamon and lemon peel, and barely cover with water. Bring to boil, cover and simmer until the berries have burst. Pour through a strainer and boil again with the sugar and a third of the butter in the rest of the water. Stir in the cornflour mixed with the wine. Cut the bread into small cubes and cook in the remaining butter until golden yellow. Use as a garnish with the mint leaves.

8–9 large elderberry clusters
1 cinnamon stick
peel of half a lemon
³/₄ cup (150g) sugar
6 tablespoons (75g) butter
salt
1 tablespoon cornflour
¹/₂ cup red wine
6 cups (1 ¹/₂ litres) water
4 slices toasted bread with crust removed
mint leaves

Salads

FENNEL SALAD WITH LEMON SAUCE

2 fennel bulbs
1 onion
3 small pickled cucumbers,
*   gherkins or cornichons*
1 hard-boiled egg
¹/₂ tablespoon capers
¹/₂ teaspoon peppermint leaves
4 tablespoons oil
3 tablespoons lemon juice
pinch of salt

Fennel is highly prized for aiding digestion. Remove the fennel from the hard, external rind, and cut in half. Place in salt water for about 15 minutes. Cut the stalks into eighths and sprinkle with a little of the lemon juice. To prepare the lemon sauce, cut the other ingredients into small pieces and mix with the oil and the rest of the lemon juice. Add 2–3 tablespoons of vegetable stock if the sauce is too thick. Place a small glass containing the lemon sauce in the middle of a serving plate and surround with the fennel pieces. Garnish the salad with sprigs of watercress.

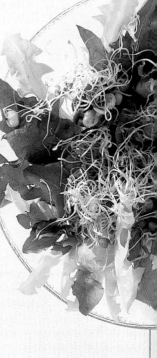

SALAD WITH THREE WILD HERBS

3oz (75g) equal parts yarrow,
*   plantain and watercress*
*   leaves*
a little garlic, to taste
half a cucumber
freshly chopped or dried chives
*   and parsley*
1 medium, boiled cold potato
salad dressing consisting of
*   lemon and cream, or lemon*
*   and oil*

Yarrow stimulates metabolism. Plantain leaves are rich in mucilage and have anti-inflammatory properties. Wash the herbs carefully and allow to drain. Cut the yarrow and plantain into fine strips. Cube cucumber and potato into small pieces. Leave watercress whole and arrange in bowl. Add herbs and other vegetables and salad dressing and mix well.

CHICORY SALAD

¹/₂ lb (250g) chicory
1 banana
3 oranges
1 tablespoon lemon juice
1 tablespoon Dijon mustard
1 teaspoon sugar
¹/₂ cup cream, beaten thick
3 tablespoons roasted
*   almonds*
salt, pepper

Cut the chicory, the banana and the oranges into fine slices, and place the slices in alternating layers on a plate. Sprinkle with a dash of salt and sugar, and add the lemon juice and the mustard. Carefully spoon the cream around and underneath the layers and garnish with slivered, lightly roasted almonds.

DANDELION SALAD

¹/₂ cup young dandelion greens
2 cups lettuce or spinach
¹/₂ cup alfalfa sprouts
¹/₄ cup beansprouts

Thoroughly wash the young dandelion greens. Chop and mix with lettuce and sprouts. Toss with your favourite creamy dressing and serve.

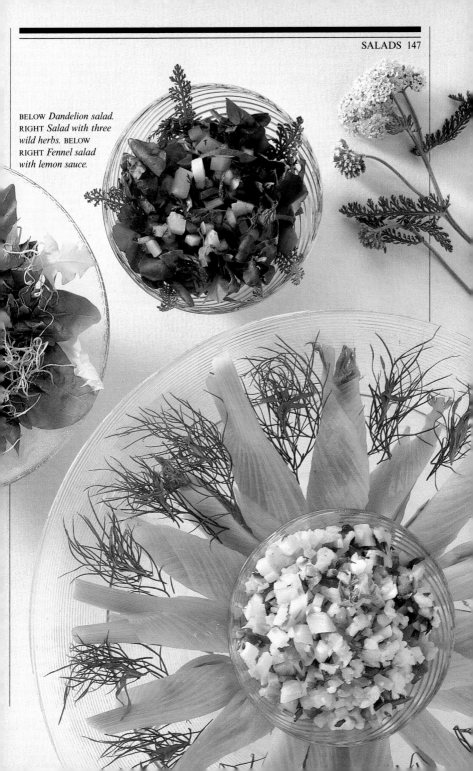

BELOW *Dandelion salad.*
RIGHT *Salad with three wild herbs.* BELOW
RIGHT *Fennel salad with lemon sauce.*

Snacks and savouries

SORREL AND PARSNIP MOUSSE WITH CARROT SAUCE (SERVES 6)

For the mousse:
1lb (450g) parsnips, peeled
and cut into large pieces
about 36 sorrel leaves
4 tablespoons (50g) butter
$\frac{1}{2}$ cup (50g) plain flour
1 cup (275ml) milk
1 egg, separated
1 tablespoon chopped chives
salt and black pepper

For the sauce:
$\frac{1}{2}$ lb carrots, peeled and
chopped
1 cup of vegetable stock
juice of 1 orange

Sorrel contains vitamin C, and is thought, like spinach, to enhance the haemoglobin content of the blood. Place the parsnips in a saucepan, with a little water, cover and simmer for 20 minutes until tender. Preheat an oven to 190°C (375°F). Quickly dip each sorrel leaf into a bowl of boiling water to blanch, and use the leaves to line the bases and sides of 6 ramekin dishes (about 6 leaves for each dish). When the parsnips are cooked, drain and mash them thoroughly. Melt the butter in a pan, add the flour and cook for 2 minutes, stirring until smooth. Gradually add the milk and simmer while stirring to make a smooth, thick sauce. Beat the egg yolk into the sauce. Whisk the egg white until soft peaks form. Mix the sauce and parsnips together, with the chives and seasoning. Fold in the egg white. Divide the mixture between the ramekin dishes. Place the dishes into a deep roasting tin half filled with hot water. Bake for 50 minutes until the mousses turn puffy. Turn out and serve while they are still hot.

For the sauce, boil the carrots in the stock until soft then blend in a food processor. Add the orange juice and season to taste. Reheat to serve and garnish with chopped chives.

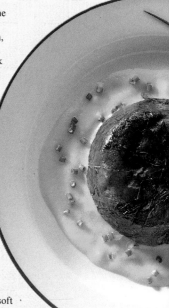

CREAMED WATERCRESS LOAF (SERVES 4)

3 cups watercress
4 hard-boiled eggs, finely
chopped
1 cup (275ml) thick or double
cream
$\frac{1}{2}$ cup breadcrumbs
salt and pepper

Watercress is rich in iron (which is necessary for the formation of haemoglobin) and is widely considered good for the blood. Steam the watercress for 5 minutes, drain and season to taste. Preheat an oven to 180°C (350°F). Thoroughly mix the watercress, eggs and breadcrumbs. Pour into a greased loaf pan. Pour in the cream, cutting the mixture with a knife so the cream penetrates well. Bake for 30 minutes, or until firm. Serve while still hot.

ABOVE *Sorrel and parsnip mousse, served in a carrot sauce.*

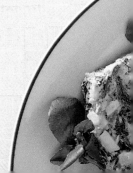

LEFT *Fresh pasta, a good energy food, high in carbohydrates, can be served simply, tossed in olive oil with various fresh herbs, including parsley and fennel (aids to digestion) and oregano (which also aids digestion and helps to relieve rheumatism).*

ABOVE *Broad beans, which are rich in protein and contain some iron and vitamin B, may be served in chervil as a blood tonic and aid to digestion.*

LEFT *Creamed watercress loaf.*

Desserts

LEMON BALM SORBET (SERVES 4)

³/₄ cup (75g) caster sugar
1 cup (275ml) water
1¹/₄ cup lemon balm
juice of 1 lemon
1 egg white

Lemon balm is famous as a relaxant. This sorbet can also be made with mint (which is an anti-flatulent and a gentle stimulant) or rosemary (which improves the digestion and is good for high blood pressure). Place the sugar in a saucepan and pour on the water. Bring to the boil, stirring, until the sugar is dissolved. Chop the lemon balm and add to the pan. Cover the pan and remove it from the heat. Leave to infuse for 20–30 minutes. Test for flavour, and if it is not intense enough, bring it to the boil again and leave to infuse for a further 15 minutes. Strain the liquid and add the lemon juice. Transfer the mixture to a freezer tray and freeze for 2–3 hours. When the sorbet is only partly frozen, whisk the egg white until stiff and fold it into the mixture. Return to the freezer for a further 3–4 hours or until frozen. Serve the sorbet in individual dishes and decorate each serving with extra leaves of the herb.

DANDELION FRITTERS (SERVES 4)

4 cups dandelion flowers
¹/₂ cup vegetable oil
1 cup milk
1 cup biscuit mix
1 tablespoon honey

Dandelion tops have been used as a treatment for liver ailments. Mix together the biscuit mix, milk and honey. Heat the oil in a pan until it sizzles when a little of the mixture is dropped into it. Dip the dandelion flowers in the mixture and drop them head first into the hot oil. Fry until golden brown. Turn over with a spoon and brown the other side. Remove and drain the fritters on kitchen paper before serving.

GOOSEBERRY AND ELDERFLOWER SOUFFLE (SERVES 4)

1lb (500g) gooseberries
1 stripped head of elderflower
4 tablespoons vanilla sugar
4 eggs, separated
¹/₂ cup (140ml) lightly whipped cream
1 tablespoon (15g) gelatine

Elderflowers soothe respiratory problems, including hay fever. Gently poach the gooseberries in the water with the elderflowers and 3 tablespoons of vanilla sugar. Strain off the juice and strain the fruit. Dissolve the gelatine in a few spoonfuls of the warm gooseberry juice. Whisk the egg yolks with the remaining sugar until thick and pale, then mix them into the fruit purée with the cream and gelatine. Leave it for 10 minutes for the mixture to thicken. Whisk the egg whites until stiff, and fold them into the purée mixture. Pour the mixture into a soufflé dish and leave to set in a cool place.

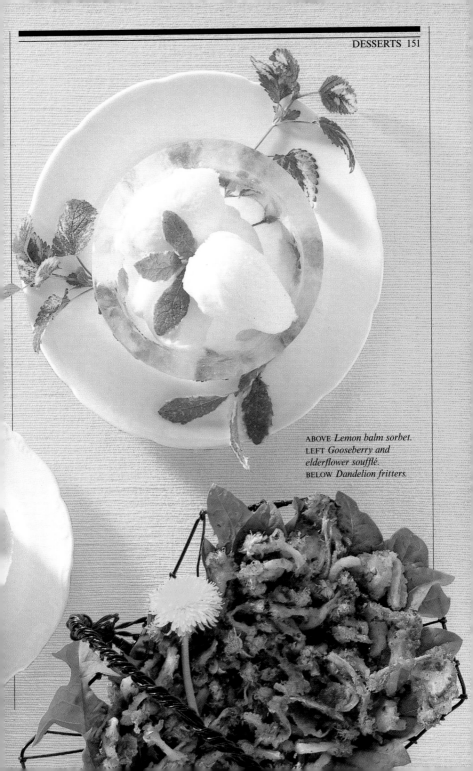

ABOVE *Lemon balm sorbet.*
LEFT *Gooseberry and
elderflower soufflé.*
BELOW *Dandelion fritters.*

Bread and biscuits

HERB BREAD

4 cups flour
1 oz (25g) yeast
³/₄ cup milk
1 egg
2 tablespoons shortening
¹/₄ cup water
2 tablespoons sugar
1 teaspoon salt
2 teaspoons caraway seeds
¹/₂ teaspoon sage
¹/₂ teaspoon nutmeg

Caraway improves the digestion, and sage is an excellent general source of vitality. Dissolve the yeast in the water. Heat the milk until it is simmering. Add the sugar, shortening and salt. Leave until lukewarm and beat in the egg, seasoning, nutmeg, caraway seed and sage. Add to the yeast. Add 2 cups of sifted flour and beat until smooth. Add enough of the remaining flour to make a soft dough. Turn out onto a lightly floured board and knead until elastic. Shape into a ball and place in a greased bowl, turning the dough to grease it all over. Cover with a cloth and allow to rise in a warm place until the dough has doubled in size (this should take about 1 hour). Punch down and allow to stand for a further 10 minutes. Shape into a round loaf and place in a greased round pan. Cover and allow to rise again for about 1 hour. Bake at 200°C (400°F) for 45 minutes or until brown. Brush with melted shortening.

PARSLEY AND BACON BREAD

4 cups (¹/₂ kg) flour
4 teaspoons baking powder
1 teaspoon salt
1 egg
1 cup (275 ml) milk
2 tablespoons (30g)
  margarine
2 tablespoons chopped parsley
3 slices bacon, finely chopped
a little milk for glazing

Parsley helps improve digestion. Beat the egg and add to the milk. Sift in the flour and salt. Melt the margarine and add to the mixture. Mix in the parsley and bacon and form a dough. Shape into two small or one large loaf and place on a greased baking sheet. Brush with the milk and bake at 215°C (425°F) for about 30–35 minutes.

CHAMOMILE AND LAVENDER BREAD

4 cups (¹/₂ kg) flour
4 teaspoons baking powder
1 teaspoon salt
1 egg
1 cup (275ml) milk
1 cup (275ml) chamomile
  infusion
2 tablespoons (30g)
  margarine
2 tablespoons lavender
  flowers

Chamomile infusion has calming and tonic effects. Beat the egg. Add to the milk and the infusion. Add the lavender. Sift in the flour and salt, with the melted margarine. Form a dough and place on a greased tray. Bake at 215°C (425°F) for 30 minutes.

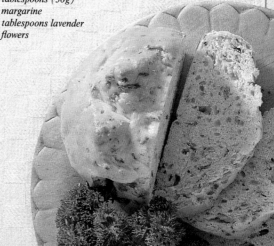

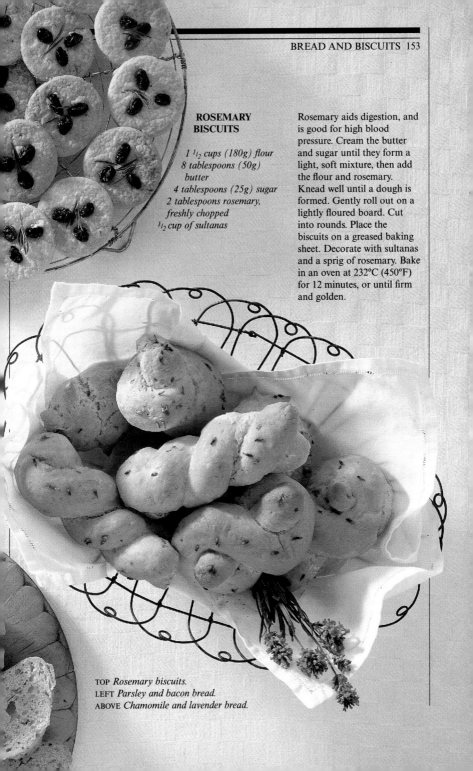

ROSEMARY BISCUITS

1 1/2 cups (180g) flour
8 tablespoons (50g)
butter
4 tablespoons (25g) sugar
2 tablespoons rosemary,
freshly chopped
1/2 cup of sultanas

Rosemary aids digestion, and is good for high blood pressure. Cream the butter and sugar until they form a light, soft mixture, then add the flour and rosemary. Knead well until a dough is formed. Gently roll out on a lightly floured board. Cut into rounds. Place the biscuits on a greased baking sheet. Decorate with sultanas and a sprig of rosemary. Bake in an oven at 232°C (450°F) for 12 minutes, or until firm and golden.

TOP *Rosemary biscuits.*
LEFT *Parsley and bacon bread.*
ABOVE *Chamomile and lavender bread.*

Cosmetics and bathing

Many cosmetic preparations can be made from plants found in the garden and the countryside. Lotions made of lemon juice, lily-of-the-valley flowers and witch hazel soften and tighten the skin, while woodruff, lime or linden flowers and potato juice not only soften and tone the skin but also remove wrinkles. Ground sunflower seeds with some water make an excellent nourishing pore cleanser. Apple and avocado pulp also nourish the skin when used as a night cream, and lotions or cold creams prepared from almond and coconut oils are both soothing and protective. Among the most common natural cosmetics are slices of cucumber or tomato placed on the face to tighten the pores and freshen the eyes.

An infusion of red clover or elder

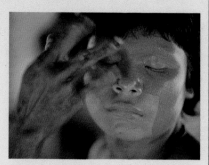

The use of some form of cosmetic is an almost universal human trait. This Amazonian Xingu is having her face painted with tree-bark extract.

flowers heals skin made sore by the sun and wind, and golden rod leaves, mullein flowers or watercress can be boiled in milk to yield a soothing complexion milk. Mixtures of peppermint,

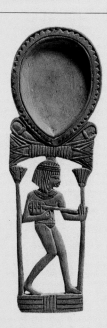

An Egyptian ointment spoon, c.1580–1080BC.

PERFUMES

The ancient Egyptians were expert perfume makers, and the guilds of ointment perfumers of Israel and other Near Eastern nations were the precursors of the present-day apothecaries. The non-Spartan Greeks were great lovers of perfumes, which they began to use on a lavish scale following Alexander's conquest of Egypt in 330BC. Similarly, the Roman conquest of Persia and the Middle East ushered in the use of rose oils and other perfumes by Roman matrons.

The distillation of alcohol was discovered in the 4th century BC, and around AD1000 the Arab physician Avicenna first distilled the essential oil or attar of rose. The art of distillation made Arabia the centre for the production and export of perfumes extracted from raw materials which were often imported from China, India or Tibet. Perfumes and essences were reintroduced to Europe in AD1200 by the returning Crusaders. The independent discovery of the distillation of attar of roses in Ravenna in AD1574 led to France becoming the centre for perfume making in Europe. In the late 19th century, natural perfumes began to be replaced by synthetic terpenes and other aroma chemicals.

sage, chamomile and lime or linden flowers in a bowl of boiling hot water provide an effective facial steam that softens and beautifies the skin.

Nourishing face masks and packs which stimulate circulation while cleansing and improving the texture and elasticity of the skin can be made from a variety of plants, including oats and barley, tomatoes, strawberries, bananas, apricots and peaches. Dandelion, daisy and nettle leaves make an effective face mask when mashed together, as does a strong infusion of elder flowers, mixed with yogurt.

Infusions of agrimony, chamomile, eyebright or elder flowers add sparkle to the eyes, and marigold, succory and vervain flower infusions are used to soothe tired or inflamed eyes. Infusions of rosemary or chamomile flowers, bay rum and boxwood leaves promote the growth of new hair and lemon juice, diluted in water, highlights and cleans the hair after shampooing. Sunflower seeds, wheat germ and avocado produce a rich hair conditioner.

Used as a dentifrice, strawberry juice or powdered arece nut charcoal whitens the teeth, removes tartar and sweetens the breath. Alfalfa, horseradish, liquorice or marshmallow roots, soaked in warm water to soften them, can be used as a natural tooth brush.

A definite improvement should be seen after 12 days of using herbal skin cleansers and other plant-based beauty treatments. Since the condition of the

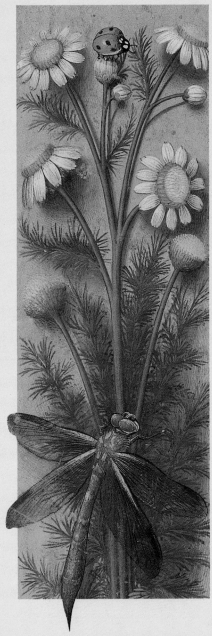

Chamomile, from the Book of Hours *commissioned by Anne of Britanny (1477–1514). A decoction of chamomile and rosemary flowers provides a refreshing, oily skin toner, skin cleanser and hair rinse.*

skin is dependent upon the health of the body, the use of herbal treatments for skin conditions is best complemented by eating uncooked salads of dandelion, parsley and yarrow leaves. Supplementary teas – made of the same plant that is being used on the skin – and a one-day fruit and vegetable diet cleanse the body and boost the action of the cosmetic treatment.

The human skin carries out the vital functions of respiration, protecting the

CLEANLINESS

The ancient Israelites emphasized strict hygiene, washing and bathing in fresh water. Most cultures had a more luxurious approach to bathing. Egyptian women bathed in scented waters and both sexes rubbed aromatic bath ointments into their skin. The Greeks bathed in aromatic oils and wet steam baths, and the Romans washed with rose water and liberally used lavender as an aromatic in their daily baths. Roman thermal baths contained pipes of scented waters and, with a capacity for 2,000 bathers, were the centre of Roman social life. The Arabs washed themselves daily in public baths of which there were 2,000 in medieval Baghdad alone. Public baths were also a part of popular culture in medieval Europe.

The use of dry-heat vapour baths for hygiene and medicine extended from Central America northward to the Eskimo and through northern Eurasia into Ireland. The Mayas used vapour sweatbaths in

childbirth and for treating colds, rheumatism and other ailments. The hot spring baths of Japan, where bathing is a highly developed art form, the French centres for thalassotherapy, which use algae and warm seawater, and the continental spas are all aspects of an international therapeutic complex of ideas centred around bathing.

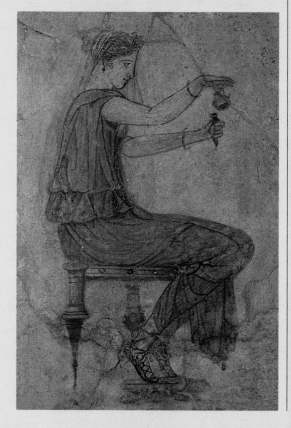

In this wall painting from the Villa Farnesina in Rome, c.50BC, a girl pours a bath scent into a small vase.

body from toxins, regulating the body's temperature and eliminating waste materials. Water is an essential means of keeping the skin clean and healthy, and the refreshing and strengthening effects of a full warm bath can be enhanced by the addition of plant or plant-derived materials, which stimulate and relax the body and tonify the skin. An infusion or decoction of plant material may be poured into a warm bath or used to fill a small bag or clean stocking, which is then hung underneath the hot tap when filling the tub.

The addition of pine, larch and other coniferous sprouts relieves tension and strain and stimulates the nerves, blood circulation and skin metabolism. Camphor, eucalyptus and mint bath additives also have a salutary effect on blood circulation. The regular use of horse chestnut extract vitalizes skin tissue and metabolism, and supports venous circulation in the legs, particularly during and after pregnancy.

Rosemary, juniper and lavender-flower additives have a refreshing and soothing effect on the nervous system. Valerian, hop or chamomile additives promote a sound night's sleep and mugwort relieves fatigue and aching muscles, while hay-flower and juniper baths help soothe rheumatic ailments. Wheat bran and horsetail are good for inflamed skin, chamomile for wounds and oak bark for haemorrhoids and leucorrhoea.

For tired feet, footbaths prepared with rosemary, wild thyme or linden flowers are helpful, and hay-flower or oat-straw foot-baths

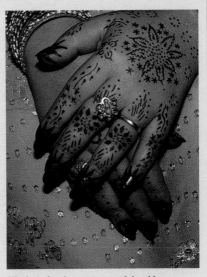

The hair dye, henna, is one of the oldest cosmetics known, having been used to paint fingernails, hands and feet since before the time of Cleopatra. It is prepared from the henna shrub of Iran, India and Africa.

are beneficial in treating open wounds, sweating feet and other foot ailments. After a foot-bath, the feet and legs should be rubbed with olive oil impregnated with marigold petals. Essential oil drops can also be used as bath additives to keep the skin soft and supple, relaxing the muscles, and replenishing the body's natural oils. Rosemary, peppermint and pine oils have a stimulating effect; lemon balm, sage and lavender oils are relaxing, and olive oil with apricot or cucumber juice is recommended for dry skin.

Soap-nuts, which yield a rich lather when rubbed in water, are used as a soap-substitute in Tanzania.

Aromatherapy

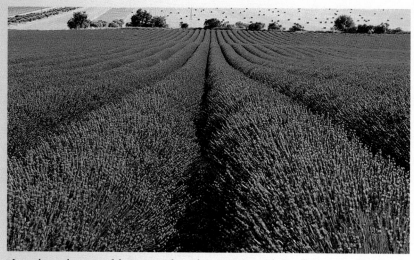

Lavender produces one of the most popular and aromatic essential oils, which is an excellent remedy for insect bites and burns, as well as headaches, insomnia and circulatory problems.

Aromatherapy is a method of promoting physical and emotional well-being through the inhalation and application of essential oils that have been extracted from flowering plants. Many of the volatile oils used in aromatherapy, such as cinnamon, eucalyptus, juniper, thyme and tea tree, have antiseptic, antibacterial and anti-inflammatory properties. When inhaled, the oils' evaporated molecules are taken up by receptor cells that transmit electrochemical messages to the limbic part of the brain, which controls emotions, motivated behaviour and neuroendocrine functions. The odours of the oils evoke memories and images, alter moods, arouse sexual emotions, or exhibit calming and restorative properties. For example, bergamot, melissa, sandalwood and ylang-ylang oils all alleviate anxiety and depression.

The use of essential oils for health care and allurement is more than 4,000 years old. There are numerous biblical references to medicinal balms and holy anointing oils. The Egyptians imported large quantities of fragrant gums and resins from Arabia and India, which were processed into scented unguents, perfumes and oils by temple priests for cosmetic, medicinal and ritual purposes. The ancient Greek physician, Hippocrates, recognized the therapeutic value of plant oils and prescribed numerous fragrant oils for their soothing and stimulating properties.

Modern aromatherapists use some forty essential oils, including citrus, geranium, jasmine, lemon, patchouli and rose. These highly concentrated oils are carefully measured in drops and diluted in a base or carrier oil of cold-pressed sweet almond, olive, or other nut, seed or vegetable oils. Two or three fragrant oils may be blended with natural oils from the same botanical family or according to grouping by fragrance (herby, floral, musky and spicy). The natural anti-inflammatory potency of chamomile oil, for example, is greatly increased by adding myrrh oil in the correct proportion.

Massage, involving rubbing, kneading and stroking the body, relaxes the individual, soothes and relieves strains and muscular aches and stimulates blood circulation near the skin's surface, facilitating the entry of the oils into the body. Essential oil molecules relax and stimulate nerve endings, and are carried throughout the body by the blood and lymph. Aromatherapists utilize a variety of methods and techniques, including remedial and Swedish massage, shiatsu and reflexology. Essential oils may also be safely and enjoyably used at home as a minor first aid treatment, and to improve beauty and health. Essential oils are added to cold creams, lotions, facial masks and hair and scalp treatments. Placed in diffusers and ring burners, they bring freshness to the home and office. However, a number of essential oils, such as cinnamon, fennel and nutmeg, are unsafe for inexperienced users. Others may irritate the skin, or like myrrh, sage and rosemary, be unsafe for pregnant women.

THE BIRTH OF MODERN AROMATHERAPY

The term "aromatherapy" was coined by the French cosmetic chemist René-Maurice Gattefossé in 1928 to describe the therapeutic properties of lavender and other aromatic plant oils. Essential oils were used for healing the wounds of soldiers in World War II, and the biochemist Marguerite Maury subsequently developed the cosmetic and therapeutic methods of applying essential oils with massages.

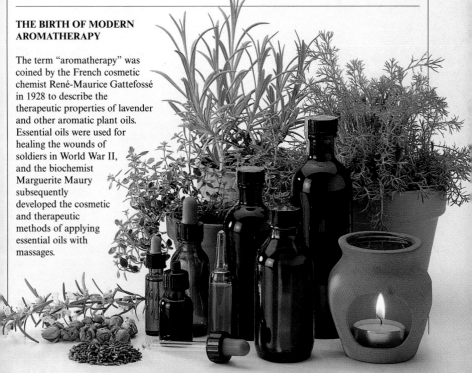

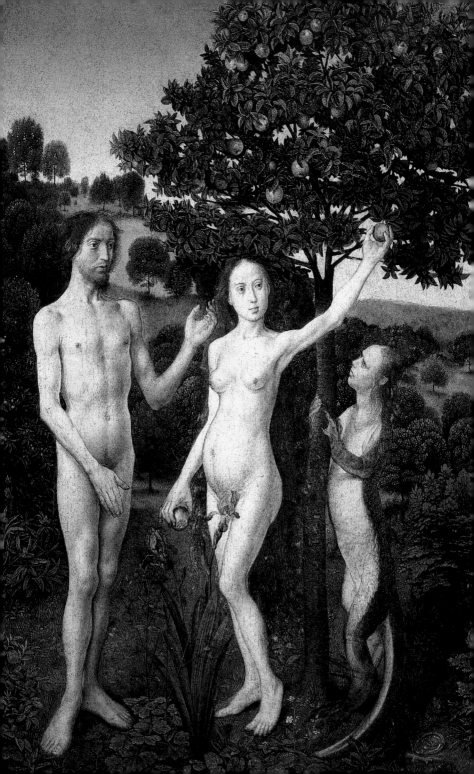

Folklore

Sacred trees and plants

Plants are not only used to heal, or prevent disease in, individual human bodies and minds. Their use in folklore and legend is a factor in the cultural well-being and cohesion of entire peoples. Trees and other plants pervade artistic and spiritual symbology, from the Tree of Liberty to the maypole and the Christmas tree. These symbolic trees embody and express the unity of all life, and provide a communication with the divine centre and source of life. In paintings, songs and stories, flowers present a face of exuberant life, but conceal the twilight of death; while the seed displays the husk of death, beneath which waits new life.

The iconographic and mythological meanings attached to trees in different cultures are vast and varied, and include well-being, sustenance and fertility, abundance, divine motherhood, the Milky Way, eternal life, nature, and the living cosmos endlessly regenerating and renewing itself. Mythic symbols can never be fully explicated, however, since the meaning within them loses its richness of implication when fully revealed. For the Maoris, Latvians and many other peoples throughout the world, forests were the favourite haunt of demons, elves, fairies, wild men, moss-wifekins and other forest spirits. By analyzing a vast collection of these beliefs and rituals concerning plants and trees, Sir James Frazer formed what one critic termed the Covent Garden or vegetable school of mythology. Frazer postulated that numerous deities were originally tree-spirits or corn demons, and that tree-worship was a universal form of religious behaviour. Deities, spirits and ancestral shades used trees as dwelling places, or depended on trees for existence. However, no living tree or wooden pillar was ever worshipped as a deity, only the divine spirit that it contained, or of which it was the ritual display.

Universal trends

Mythic images of a cosmic tree occur throughout the world and resemble one another to an extraordinary degree. The image of an inverted tree, with its roots in the sky, occurs in Austrian folk art, in Siberia, among the Makiritare of Venezuela and elsewhere. A paradisaical, milk-yielding tree which suckles child-like souls is found as far apart as ancient Egypt and Mexico. These similarities have been attributed both to parallel, independent development and to historical connections and migrations. They have even been cited as the

LEFT *Adam and Eve being tempted at the tree of the knowledge of good and evil, painted by Hugo van der Goes (1440–82).*

BELOW *Druids gathering mistletoe, from Buland's* L'histoire des papes. *Druid means "The Finder of the Oak Tree" in Celtic. Druids were the priests, teachers and judges of Celtic society; they lived in oak forests, in whose clearings they held their religious festivals, which sometimes involved human sacrifice.*

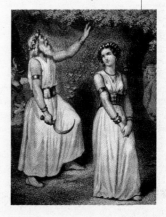

by-product of an unconscious imagery to which the human mind is biologically predisposed. However, since the tree, as an autonomous, primordial image, reflects both external, cultural and internal, psychological happenings, there can be no master key, or individual, all-inclusive theory which is elevated over the others.

Wooden posts, symbolic of the tree and associated with sacrificial animal skulls, occur as far back as the Upper Palaeolithic period (12,000BC) on the north European plain among ancient reindeer hunters, who probably possessed a shamanistic religion. The world tree is a central and universal element of the shamanic cosmos and, as an aspect of an exceedingly ancient and widespread religious phenomena, it is not surprising that it has been adapted to innumerable historical and contemporary religions.

Hallowed sites

Sacred groves occur throughout the world. In them, no wood may be cut or firewood gathered, and no animal hunted. In Ghana, Nigeria and other African countries, each community maintains a sacred grove, the abode of protective and ancestral spirits, in which secret initiation and other religious rites are carried out. Among the Atonga of west Africa, the sacred groves are under the jurisdiction of a sisterhood of priestesses. Any man entering a grove by accident is required to join the secret sodality and dress and live like a woman for the rest of his life. In India, sacred groves were the first temples of divine worship and are still religiously preserved in many areas. Annual festivals as well as personal prayers and sacrifices are carried out there. Up to 49 acres (20ha) in extent, they are the last remnants of the virgin monsoon forests, and function as a preserve for animals, as well as for rare orchids and other plants of medicinal value. The Karen and Akha of Thailand conduct New Year ceremonies in their sacred groves at which sacrificial offerings are presented to the spirit-owners of the trees.

The Greeks and Romans used to build walled temple sanctuaries (*sacellum*) around their fig groves. Sacred groves also occur in Syria, Turkey, Sri Lanka, Burma, southern China, Samoa and other Pacific Islands. They were centres of religious and political life for Germanic, Slavic and Finno-Ugaric tribes. In 11th-century Lithuania, Christians were not permitted to approach sacred groves because they would contaminate them. In the Middle Ages, these groves were royal forests: the king's hunting preserves and sanctuaries for criminals.

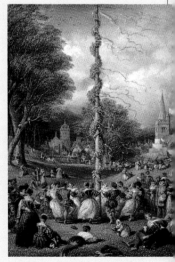

Maypole dances take place throughout Europe, as well as in India and Latin America. They are relics of ancient fertility dances, which were originally conducted around a living tree.

Near East and Europe

In the story of Genesis there are two trees, the tree of eternal life and the tree of the knowledge of good and evil, with its forbidden fruit. The Bible concludes with the vision of a New Jerusalem in which the tree of life bears leaves for the healing of nations. Babylonian myth also had a tree of life and a tree of truth, guarding the entrance to heaven. The sacred date palm and waterlily of Egypt were incorporated into their architectural column-capitals and later adapted in Doric and Ionian pillars to represent the life tree. Both the life tree (*tuba*) of Sassanian-Arabian art and the Jewish seven-branched seferotic tree of light are inverted; rooted in heaven and extending downward to express the divinity's descent into humanity. Recollections of the life tree became interwoven with medieval traditions of the tree of the cross, whose roots pierced down to hell and whose top reached to heaven. In apocryphal texts, the cross of Christ was made of a tree which had sprung from the tree of knowledge in Eden.

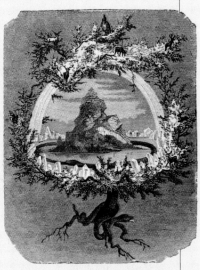

People from plants

The Greeks believed that Zeus created a race of men from the trunk of a cosmogonic ash tree and, in Norse myth, dwarfs fashioned the first human pair, Ash and Elm, out of trees. According to Celtic folklore, the first man sprang from an elder, the first woman from a mountain-ash. In Belgium, England, France and Italy, a tree is planted in the garden on the birth of a child. In German-speaking countries an apple tree is planted for a boy and a pear tree for a girl. (Apples were also once placed in the hand of a child when he or she was buried, "to play with in Paradise". This practice may relate to myths of the golden apples of the garden of Hesperides and the apples of Idun, which were long believed to give immortality.) Until recently, in Europe and the US, a small child would be passed through a cleft oak or ash tree as a cure for hernia or rickets.

In Europe on the morning of a wedding day the bride and bridegroom may plant a pair of oaks or bushes near the house. As long as the tree lasts, the memory and influence of the event will be kept alive. In the US and Europe, contractors will often place a live tree on top of a building to celebrate the completion of a new dwelling. Termed "topping out", the practice harks back to a time when the ridge pole, which joined all the roof rafters, was the closest to heaven, and the tacked-on tree served as an offering to the gods in return for approval of the dwelling.

The Norse great ash tree, Yggdrasil, represented the universe and rose, evergreen and glittering with dew, above the hall of the three Norns of the past, present and future. Its branches stretched out over heaven and earth and under its three roots were Hel, the cold land of torture, the land of the frost-giants and the realm of humans. Under its shadow the gods assembled daily to dispense justice and make laws. The fire of a demon will burn the tree at the end of the world, but it will be renewed again, fair and green, and the gods will once more congregate under its branches.

Africa

The Sandawe, Fon, Subiya, Nuer and other African peoples believe that the first humans emerged from a cosmic tree. The first man and woman of the Zulu and Thonga emerged from a reed stalk created by God, and the Yao and Makonde generalize this concept in having the first humans coming out of bushes or a dense tropical forest. At the inauguration of Baganda kings, sacred bark cloth trees were ceremoniously planted and carefully tended, since their flourishing growth was inextricably connected to the life and power of the king.

Birth and death

Many African peoples plant a life tree upon the birth of a child. The Gesu plant two trees near the door of their homes as a residence for the good spirit which protects the child. Waadshagga parents plant a cultivated food plant, related to their clan, with the child's umbilical cord. The Swahili bury a newborn baby's placenta and umbilical cord in the courtyard and 7 days later plant a coconut palm with the child's hair and nail clippings at the same place. The palm tree is considered as the navel of the child, who is linked with the life and well-being of the plant.

The Yaka of Zaire imagine a macrocosmic womb in the form of a raffia palm tree suspended between heaven and earth, which provides for the ever-renewed generation of life. In a Yaka gynaecological healing ritual, the macrocosmic significance of the raffia palm tree is transferred to the patient's body. The foot of the sacred palm tree designates patrilineal ancestry, the tree top the living descendants of the ancestors and the right and left branches agnatic descent and uterine filiation, respectively. In these ritual contexts, tangled vines represent negative forces, sorcery and illness.

Renowned Yaka medical practitioners are buried in a foetal position with an inflorescence of the parasol tree on the head in order to ensure a rapid rebirth. African chiefs and kings are often buried in or under sacred trees. The Wolof place the bodies of their revered singers and drummers upright in hollowed-out sacred trees and the Mandingo people plant three sacred baobab trees over the head, navel and feet of their mighty hunters and famous heroes.

Forms of initiation

The mudyi tree (*Diplorrhyncus condylocarpon*), which exudes a milky-white latex, is a key symbol in the girls' puberty rite of the Ndembu people of Zambia. The mudyi tree is a many-layered symbol representing female breasts and milk, nourishment, the slender suppleness of the initiates, the mother–child bond, the Ancestress, motherhood, women's

For the Mbuti Pygmies of the equatorial rainforest, song is a potent means of communicating with the Forest and its bountiful Lord. The breath of the singers, linked to the spirit within them, directs their hopes to the Forest, which is the centre of spirit power.

In Nigeria, trees and forests are also the abode of diminutive spirit beings, who are given offerings to ward off evil. These spirits are the Owners of the Animals, and instruct humans in the use of magical medicines prepared from plants.

wisdom, matriliny, death and suffering, and the unity and continuity of Ndembu society. Each symbolic aspect becomes dominant in a specific episode of the ritual.

Eboka (*Tabernanthe iboga*), a member of the dogbane family, is a flowering shrub native to the equatorial rainforest of west-central Africa. Containing ibogaine and eleven other related alkaloids, eboka is used to treat impotence, frigidity, infertility and for endurance in hunting. It is also employed as a hallucinogen by the Bwiti and other religious movements of Gabon, Cameroon and the Congo. According to the Bwiti religion, the eboka plant arose from the flesh of a Pygmy dismembered by the creator god. By consuming it, devotees obtain new life and come to terms with death by becoming conscious of their souls' universal existence.

Small amounts of eboka are taken in order to be able to sing, dance and drum throughout rigorous Bwiti ceremonies, but to become initiated into the religion, individuals take massive doses, once or twice in their lifetimes. Initiation begins with a song and dance cycle before midnight, which celebrates creation, birth and the spirits' arrival from the land of the dead. The initiates are administered a small dose of eboka to ascertain whether they are worthy of receiving Bwiti, the divine, universal ancestor. The next morning each initiate begins to ingest the sacred plant, under the supervision of two monitors, and in the afternoon is taken from the temple to a forest stream for confession and ritual cleansing. The Fang, who consider Bwiti to be the religion of the forest, then rub the novice down with the bark of twelve sacred trees. In the temple, the initiate continues to eat eboka and at midnight collapses or "dies", allowing the soul to fly on the path of birth and death. The initiate may return to his or her prenatal existence, hear the voices of deceased relatives or, more commonly, be escorted by a spirit-guide through a deep forest to the village of the ancestral spirits, who open the door to the divinity. Toward morning, the congregation falls silent, except for the strings of the sacred harp, whose melodies are the voice of the sister of god. The initiates recount their experiences and partake of a communal meal.

Dutch scientists are testing ibogaine as a treatment for heroin and cocaine addictions. Within therapeutic settings, it unleashes repressed, childhood memories of the problems that may have helped form an addictive personality. Through reliving these experiences visually and emotionally, addicts reassess their lives. Ibogaine interacts with the dopamine neurotransmitters that play a role in drug-abuse disorders, and the waking dreams elicited by the drug may break up the brain circuitry laid down when the addiction was acquired.

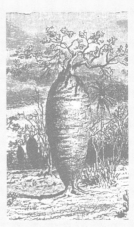

In Nigeria, the sacred tree or pole represents the Supreme Being. In addition, for the Ibo the cotton tree (above) is the symbol of the Earth-goddess, the creator deity and spouse of the Supreme Being. The Earth-goddess of the Idibio also lives in cotton trees and bestows animals and humans with life and growth. Other deities and ancestral spirits reside in special sacred trees and are presented offerings, sacrifices and prayers.

Asia and the Pacific

In India a vast number of plant and tree species are held in reverence and used in marriage ceremonies and other religious functions. Numerous Indian myths and iconographic motifs link trees with *yakshinis*: voluptuous female nymphs and spirits, such as Durga, the lady of the forest. The banyan tree is sacred to Brahma, Shiva and Kali, and the amaloka tree is the incarnation of Vishnu. The cosmic fig tree, Asvattha, represents eternal life and the endless cycle of birth, suffering and death. Meditation under trees is widely held to elevate the human heart, the most famous example being the Buddha, who achieved enlightenment under a bodhi tree. In China, the cosmic tree stands at the centre of the universe, and evergreen cypress and pine trees are planted on graves to strengthen the souls of the deceased and to save their bodies from corruption.

The tree of life is an essential element in central and northern Asian cosmology and ritual. Growing on a mountain at the navel of the world, its crown pierces the many-storeyed heavenly spheres. In Vedic ritual, a person making a sacrifice would climb an offering post representing the tree, and Siberian Yakut shamans similarly climb a post or birch tree to indicate their ecstatic ascent to the realm of the gods.

The first foods

Asia and the Pacific are perhaps the earliest sources for the widespread archetypal myths in which food plants grow from the dead body of a human or a god. The Ceramese Islanders of Indonesia tell of a young maiden who was sacrificed and buried during an annual festival. Her father dug up the corpse and cut it into pieces, which he reburied. From these body parts grew Indonesia's tuberous food plants. Kava is one of the most important ritual plants throughout the Pacific, and in one Tongan myth the kava rose from the head of a girl killed by her parents to feed a visiting chief. The girl was a leper, which is why the drinking of too much kava results in grey and scaly, leprous skin. According to the Marind-anim of New Guinea, kava sprang from the shoulder hairs of a stork-demon, whose legs are similar to the knotty stems of the plant. One of the most important and useful plants throughout the Pacific is the coconut. In Polynesian accounts, the first two coconut trees sprang from the buried brain of a giant eel, Te Tuna, the lord of the ocean, who was killed by Maui the semi-divine trickster hero, in a battle over Hina, a beautiful sky goddess. When the nut is husked, the Polynesians always find on it the two eyes and mouth of Te Tuna. In Bali, Java and the central Celebes, a coconut tree is planted with the afterbirth of a newborn child.

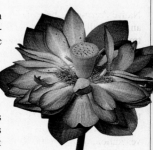

The aquatic lotus represents the female generative organ of the benevolent, universal mother goddess, Lakshmi, the womb of creation and the seat of divinity and spiritual power. In Tantric yoga, lotus symbolism is extended to the centres of the body, which correspond to particular deities and aspects of the macrocosm.

In Buddhism, the lotus rising out of the mud and water stands for the gradual attainment of transcendental wisdom out of the muddy realm of greed, hatred and delusion.

North America

Native Americans believed that an unseen spiritual power animated all natural forms, and showed great reverence for trees and flowering plants. According to the Ojibwa, all trees had souls, and for this reason they seldom cut down green or living trees, believing that it put them in great pain. The Dakota conceived of flowers as the songs of Mother Earth, and they had their own stories and songs for most of the plants they were familiar with. Each species had its own particular song which was the expression of its life and soul.

Frequently, important medicinal plants received religious veneration. The western yew, the source of an important anti-carcinogenic drug, was sacred to the Hoh and Quileute, because Great Bear, Little Bear and all the animals of the starry vault ascended from the earth on an arrow shot from a bow of yew wood. Shuswap women could not have sexual intercourse while gathering or cooking the roots and fruits of *Balsamorhiza sagittata*, an analgesic and vulnerary aid. Ginseng, an Ojibwa analgesic, was reputedly given to a youth in a trance journey to the chief of the underworld.

The flesh and the seed

Upon a child's birth, some Native Americans placed the placenta in a tree with prayers for the infant's vitality, cut the umbilical cord over an ear of corn, which was then sown and cultivated as a sacred thing, or planted a small tree which presaged the well-being of the growing child. The Mandan, Omaha and Shoshone-Crow all had ceremonies in which a cottonwood pole was erected and sung to, danced to or offered gifts as a symbol of the Great Spirit, the creation of the universe and the growth of life. Trees also had an important role in Native American death ceremonies. The Eastern Algonkians planted young maple trees, whose autumnal leaves glow like embers, over their graves, and many other groups either placed their dead in trees or, like the Nootka and Southern Kwakiutl, put the body in a wooden box, which was then placed high in a tree.

In the Wyandot creation myth, Sky Chief uproots the celestial tree and pushes his pregnant wife into the hole of the sky dome. She falls to earth and gives birth to a daughter who, in turn, dies giving birth to twin boys. Her body is buried, and from it emerge maize, pumpkins and beans. In a Cherokee myth, the first maize plants issue from the blood of an old woman killed by her disobedient and unnatural sons, and according to the Papago, coyote tobacco sprang from the grave of a murdered grandmother. In all versions of this archetypal myth, the birth of a life-giving plant necessarily proceeds out of death, murder or a primordial sacrifice.

To many peoples the tenacious, enduring cedar tree – Grandmother Cedar – was the home of the thunder-deity and the most sacred of plants. Cedar twigs are sprinkled as incense upon fires at the beginning of councils and sacred tribal rites, and the aromatic smoke is offered in sacred pipes to the six directions of Native American cosmology. A sacred cedar pole was carried by the Choctaw and Dakota in advance of the people as they moved from place to place.

The branches of the luminous Algonkian and Iroquois world tree pierce the sky and its roots extend to the waters of the underworld. Great Face, an invisible giant, guards the tree and, as chief of the Iroquois False Face Society, rubs his turtle-shell rattle upon the tree to obtain its power, which he imparts to the masks worn by the society members. They in turn rub their rattles on pine trunks in order to become imbued with sky and earth power. The cosmic world tree is richly developed in the mythology and totem poles of the Salish and other northwest-coast peoples.

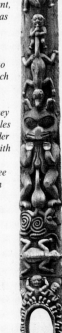

Central America

The art and literature of the ancient Mexicans, their flower festivals and the guild-like societies formed by Aztec horticulturists and florists, all attest to the importance of plants in Central America. Aztec warriors fought "flower wars" and enormous quantities of fresh flowers were brought daily to the Aztec capital for the decoration of temples, for use in dances and for the personal use of the nobility. The calendrical day sign, Flower, was dedicated to Xochiquetzal, the goddess of flowers, love and courtesans, who with her consort, Five Flower, was honoured at festivals held at the beginning, during and at the end of the rainy season.

The structure of the universe

At each corner of the mesoamerican universe stood a world tree, accompanied by a particular colour, bird, deity and unit of time. At the centre or Middle Place was a fifth tree, whose roots plunged into the watery underworld and whose branches reached, through successive heavens, to the celestial zenith. This cosmic tree connected the three worlds and served as a passageway by which the deities and spirits of the dead ascended to the highest heaven. The species of the four cosmic trees varies according to region and culture.

The representation of the world tree as a tau cross occurs in several codices and in a remarkable trilogy of tables at Palenque. Throughout the Mexican countryside are trees resembling crosses, where money and votive offerings are placed as alms for recovery from illness. The Mixe of Oaxaca sacrifice fowl under revered, cruciform trees. At the birth of a child, both the Huichol and Mixe plant a young tree, which is linked with the life and growth of the child. Aztec children who died before reaching the age of reason went to a paradisaical garden where they awaited rebirth, suckling on the milk of a great Tree of the Mother's Breast.

The rain deities of the Pipil in El Salvador are the lords of all the flowers, and lie in a marshy lake covered with mythic blue flowers which never sleep and are able to revive the dead. Cihuacoatl, the Aztec goddess of death and new life, embodies the evergreen Montezuma cypress, a funereal tree symbolic of regeneration and new life. Tamoanchan, the "place of flowers" and highest heaven of the Aztecs, is frequently depicted as a split tree with flowing streams of jewelled blood. At the beginning of time, the tree was shattered, rupturing heaven and earth and introducing time, suffering and death, as a consequence of Cihuacoatl "plucking the tree's flowers" by committing illicit sex and incest, whereupon she and her siblings were expelled from heaven.

In Xibalba, the Mayan underworld, stood a calabash tree which plays a central role in the Quiché epic, the Popol Vuh. According to this legend, a maiden wanted to taste the forbidden fruit of the tree, but the gourd she snatched spat in her hand, thereby impregnating her; whereupon she gave birth to the sun and moon. Similarly, the Pipil of El Salvador believe their rain deities to have arisen from the fruit of this tree.

The Zapotec claimed descent from cypresses and palms, to which they burned incense and gave votive offerings. The Chiapanec are said to have sprung from the roots of a ceiba tree and the ancestors of the Tzotzil and Tzeltal of Chiapas emerged from the earth through the roots of this tree. Two miraculous ceiba trees, whose leaves mingled in a spring, were transformed, upon touching earth, into the lineage ancestors of the Mixtec of Oaxaca, as shown in this illustration from a pre-Colombian Mixtec codex.

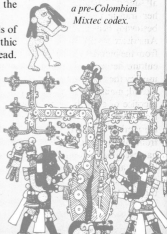

South America

The world tree which sustains and mediates heaven and earth for Amazonian peoples is the guaiac tree according to the Muisca, the moriche palm among the Warao, the wild cinnamon tree among the Mapuche, the peach palm for the Bora and Huitoto and the silk cotton tree among the Shipibo-Conibo and Mataco. The Mbyá-Guaraní have an eternal, paradisaical pindó palm at the earth's centre and four other palms at the cardinal directions, associated with various deities and winds. Among the Panare and Canelos Quichua, the centre post of their communal dwelling is a world axis, representing the cosmic tree.

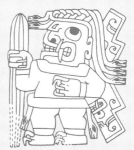

*A relief panel from the Chavin culture of northern Peru, c.1000BC. The panel shows a deity holding a San Pedro cactus (*Trichocereus pachanoi*), a hallucinogenic plant used in Chavin rituals.*

Defining spirits

The medicinal and toxic properties of plants are attributed to the spirit which resides in them. The widespread preparation of curare, an arrow poison, entails fasting, seclusion and magical songs in order to subdue the evil spirit of the plant and to develop the plant's power for cultural ends. Manioc, sweet potatoes, beans and pumpkins have, according to the Jívaro, female souls and are cultivated and prepared by the women. Maize, plantain and poisonous or intoxicating plants have male souls and may only be planted by the men. Since cotton has a male soul, Jívaro men do the spinning and weaving. In preparation for marriage, Jívaro women are given ministrations of tobacco syrup, which imbues them with the power of the tobacco spirit and the strength and ability to carry out their future domestic labours.

The Mbyá consider only those plants created by the supreme deity and growing in paradise to be sacred. *Maté*, widely used as a tea, originated, according to the Karió of Paraguay, as a bequest from their highest deity. By refusing all suitors, a maiden incurred the wrath of the deity, who had her transformed into the first *maté* tree, simultaneously bestowing health and strength upon the people. Most South American myths have culturally important plants issuing from the blood, flesh and bones of ancestral beings, civilizing culture heroes or forest spirits. A plant (*Paullinia* species), used by the Arawak as a fish poison, arose from the blood of a child; maize, beans and pumpkins originated in the selfless sacrifice of a Chaingang culture hero and manioc emerged from the body of a Parissi girl who, to spite her father, asked her mother to bury her alive. The cosmic paxiuba palm arose from the ashes of Yurupari, a divine culture hero. In a harvest ritual, widespread in the tropical rainforest, sacred flutes and trumpets fashioned from palm bark and embodying the essence of Yurupari are played to influence the growth and ripening of edible fruits.

Glossary

achene: a small, hard one-seeded fruit

agnatic: the ablity to trace descent from a common male ancestor, via other exclusively male ancestors

allopathy: the prevalent Western method of treating an illness, by prescribing a substance which provokes an opposite condition to the disease itself

alterative: a substance which, in certain doses, works a gradual change by promoting the usual function of different organs

anaesthetic: a substance which reduces pain by desensitizing the nerves

analgesic: a substance which relieves pain

antibiotic: a substance which destroys or arrests the growth of bacteria, viruses, and other micro-organisms

anti-carcinogenic: a substance which discourages the growth of a cancer

anti-inflammatory: a substance which relieves inflammation, when the body reacts to infection or injury by reddening, swelling or pain

anti-oxidant: a substance which stops molecular oxygen from working as an unwanted oxidizing agent or free radical (see below)

anti-scorbutic: a substance which treats scurvy

antiseptic: a substance applied to the skin to prevent infection

antispasmodic: a substance which relieves spasm or irregular and painful action of the musclesaperient: a substance tending mildly to stimulate the action of the bowels

astringent: a substance which, when applied to the body, renders the solids dense and firmer by drawing tissues together and drying up secretions

beriberi: a nervous disease affecting the extremities, marked by swelling and paralysis, which is caused by thiamine deficiency and is endemic to Asia

biennial: a plant which lives for two years

calyx: the outermost series of leaves; the sepals collectively

carcinogen: a substance which encourages the growth of cancer

carminative: a substance which expels gas from the stomach and intestines

cathartic: a substance which accelerates the action of the bowels

catkin: a deciduous, scaly spike of flowers

cultigen: a plant produced in cultivation and not known in the wild

cultivar: a single clone which is propagated vegetatively (that is, without using the specialized reproductive structures)

cytotoxic: a substance which is toxic to cells

decoction: the liquor extracted from a plant, or part of a plant, by boiling

demulcent: a soothing, moistening substance which modifies the action of acrid and stimulating matter upon the mucous membranes

dengue: a viral disease transmitted by mosquitoes

diaphoretic: a substance which promotes or causes the discharge of toxins via perspiration

diuretic: a substance which increases the flow of urine through its action upon the kidneys

emetic: a substance which causes vomiting

emmenagogue: a substance which promotes menstrual flow

emolient: a substance which, when applied to the solids of the body, renders them soft and flexible

erysipelas: a local feverish disease accompanied by intense inflammation of the skin

ethnopharmacology: the range of medicinal substances used by a particular people or race

expectorant: a substance which facilitates the excretion of mucus and phlegm

febrifuge: a medicine used to reduce fever

flatulence: a condition caused by gas accumulating in the stomach

flavonoid: a yellow plant pigment

fomentation: a warm poultice

free radicals: short-lived molecules which induce cells to release energy but, in excess, produce tissue damage

haemostatic: possessing a tendency to stop bleeding

homeopathy: the practice of treating an illness with substances that exacerbate its symptoms

hypermenorrhoea: excessive bleeding during menopause

hypotensive: possessing a tendency to reduce blood sugar

infusion: a plant extract obtained by soaking, rather than boiling

kwashiorkor: severe malnutrition of infants and children caused by a lack of protein

Latin names: The names of plants can vary even among speakers of the same language. The name "bluebell" refers to a kind of hyacinth in England, while in Scotland it refers to a campanula which in England is called harebell.

Latin names are a way of avoiding confusion, because they are the same all over the world, and they can also be important for safety. In North America, "hemlock" refers to a harmless forest tree, while in England it refers to a poisonous relative of parsley and fennel. As botanists' ideas about plant classification change, plants can sometimes be renamed and may be known for a time by an old and a new name. Every plant has a genus (or type) name, beginning with a capital letter. This is followed by a species name beginning with a small letter, which is different for each species of the type. This is sometimes followed by the name of the person who established the name (often abbreviated, as in "L." for the great Swedish naturalist Linnaeus). The name of the family to which the genus belongs may also be given in brackets. For example, *Hypericum perforatum* L. (Hypericaceae) belongs to the genus *Hypericum* and the species *perforatum*. The name was established by Linnaeus and the plant belongs to the family of Hypericaceae.

leucorrhoea: a discharge of mucous material from the vagina

leukaemia: an illness marked by the multiplication of the white blood cells known as leucocytes, which invade the bone marrow, lymph nodes and other parts of the body and suppress the production of blood

limbic system: that part of the brain bordering the brain stem, responsible for the emotions, hunger and sex

matrilineal: pertaining to descent through the mother

moxibustion: the application of herbs by a process of burning them on or near the skin

mucilage: a soothing, glutinous, complex carbohydrate compound found in some plants

nervine: calming to the nerves

ordeal poison: A poison administered as a test of a person's claim to have some special powers, innocence, or fitness to join a society or clan. Survival proves the individual's claim.

patrilineal: pertaining to descent through the father

perennial: a plant that lasts year after year, usually blossoming and fructifying annually

pharmacopoeia: an authoritative list of medicinal drugs, with their preparation and usage

pheromone: a chemical which is secreted by some animals and affects the behaviour or physiology of other animals in the same species

principle: the chemical constituent of a substance that causes its main characteristics

psychotropic: capable of affecting moods and mental activity

purgative: a strong laxative

refrigerant: any substance which reduces abnormal heat in the body

rubefacient: a substance which stimulates the vessels of the skin and increases its heat and redness

schistosomiasis: an infestation of the body with *Schistosoma* blood flukes

sedative: a substance that reduces nervous tension and may induce sleep

shaman: A ritual specialist in traditional societies who communes with spirits to effect cures, perform divinations or inflict harm. Often confused with sorcerers and witchdoctors.

soporific: a substance that produces sleep

spasmolytic: a substance that checks spasms or contractions

sprue: a tropical disease marked by flatulence, foul-smelling diarrhoea and emaciation

stimulant: a substance that speeds up the metabolism of the body

stomachic: any substance strengthening or stimulating the stomach

styptic: a substance or agent that, applied locally, arrests bleeding

sudorific: an agent that promotes perspiration

synergy: a combined action, usually more powerful or effective than the sum of the constituent individual actions

taproot: a long, fleshy storage root that grows vertically

thiamine: part of the vitamin B complex (B_1)

tincture: a medical extract in a solution of alcohol

tonic: a substance which gradually strengthens and tones the body or a part of it, or sharpens the appetite

umbel: a flat-topped or umbrella-shaped flower cluster with all the flower stalks radiating from a common-point

uterine: kin related through the mother

vermifuge: a substance that expels intestinal worms

vulnerary: a substance used to treat wounds

Bibliography

CHAPTER I: PLANTS AND PEOPLE

Crellin, John K. and Jane Philpott *Herbal Medicine, Past and Present* Duke University, Durham, 1990

Foster, Steven *Herbal Renaissance: Growing, Using and Understanding Herbs in the Modern World* Gibbs Smith, Salt Lake City, 1993

Griggs, Barbara *Green Pharmacy: A History of Herbal Medicine* Norman & Hobhouse, London, 1981

Hunt, Tony *Popular Medicine in Thirteenth-century England* Brewer, Wolfeboro, New Hampshire, USA and Cambridge, UK, 1990

Joyce, Christopher *Earthly Goods: Medicine Hunting in the Rainforest* Little, Brown and Company, Boston, 1994

Kapoor, P., U. O'D. Trotz and O. Simon (eds) *The Use of Medicinal Plants in the Pharmaceutical Industry* Commonwealth Science Council, London, 1992

Kinghorn, A. Douglas and Manuel F. Balandrin (eds) *Human Medicinal Agents from Plants* Amer. Chem. Soc., Washington DC, 1993

Klein, Richard M. *The Green World: An Introduction to Plants and People* Harper & Row, New York, 1987

Krieg, Margaret B. *Green Medicine* Rand McNally, Skokie, 1961

Mességué, Maurice *Of People and Plants* Inner Traditions, Rochester, 1991

Meyer, George G., Kenneth Blum and John G. Cull *Folk Medicine and Herbal Healing* Thomas Springfield, 1981

Rodriguez, E. *et al* "Thiarubine A, a bioactive constituent of Aspilia (Asteraceae) consumed by wild chimpanzees" in *Experientia, 41: 419–20*, 1985

Scarborough, John (ed.) *Folklore and Folk Medicines* Amer. Inst. Hist. Pharm., Madison, 1987

Steiner, Richard P. (ed.) *Folk Medicine: The Art and the Science* Amer. Chem. Soc., Washington DC, 1986

Swain, Tony (ed.) *Plants in the Development of Modern Medicine* Harvard University, Cambridge, 1972

Werbach, Melvyn R. and Michael T. Murray *Botanical Influences on Illness: A Sourcebook of Clinical Research* Third Line, Tarzana, 1994

Wijesekera, R.O.B. *The Medicinal Plant Industry* CRC, Boca Raton, 1991

CHAPTER II: HERBAL LEXICON

Bruneton, Jean (trans. Caroline K. Hatton) *Pharmacognosy, Phytochemistry, Medicinal Plants* Intercept, Andover, UK, 1995

Duke, James A. *CRC Handbook of Medicinal Plants* CRC, Boca Raton, 1985

Pahlow, Manfried (trans. Kathleen Luft) *The Healing Plants* Barron's Educational Series, Hauppauge, 1993

Tyler, Varro E. *Herbs of Choice: The Therapeutic Uses of Phytomedicinals* Haworth, Binghamton, New York, 1994

Weiss, Rudolf F. (trans. A.R. Meuss) *Herbal Medicine* Beaconsfield Press, Beaconsfield, 1988

Wichtl, Max (trans. and ed. Norman G. Bisset) *Herbal Drugs and Phytopharmaceuticals: A Handbook for Practice on a Scientific Basis* CRC, Boca Raton, 1995

CHAPTER III: HERBAL HEALING IN THE EAST

Anderson, Edward F. *Plants and People of the Golden Triangle: Ethnobotany of the Hill Tribes of Northern Thailand* Dioscorides, Portland, 1993

Bensky, Dan and Andrew Gamble *Chinese Herbal Medicine: Materia Medica* Eastland, Seattle, 1993

Brun, Viggo and Trond Schumacher *Traditional Herbal Medicine in Northern Thailand* University of California, Berkeley, 1987

Farnsworth, Norman and Nuntavan Bunyapraphatsara *Thai Medicinal Plants: Recommended for Primary Health Care System* Medicinal Plant Information Center, Bangkok, 1992

Foster, Steven and Yue Chongxi *Herbal Emissaries: Bringing Chinese Herbs to the West* Inner Traditions, Rochester, 1992

Frawley, David and Vasant Lad *The Yoga of Herbs: An Ayurvedic Guide to Herbal Medicine* Lotus, Twin Lakes, 1992

Hsu, Hung-yuan *Oriental Materia Medica: A Concise Guide* Oriental Healing Arts Institute, Long Beach, 1986

Huang, Kee Chang *The Pharmacology of Chinese Herbs* CRC, Boca Raton, 1993

Hyatt, Richard *Healing with Chinese Herbs* Healing Arts, Rochester, 1991

Jilek, W.G. and L. Jilek-Aall "The mental health relevance of traditional medicine and shamanism in refugee camps of northern Thailand" in *Curare, 13: 217–224,* 1990

Kapoor, L.D. *CRC Handbook of Ayurvedic Medicinal Plants* CRC, Boca Raton, 1990

Lad, Vasant *Ayurveda: The Science of Self-Healing* Lotus, Santa Fe, 1984

Lu, Henry C. *Chinese System of Food Cures: Prevention and Remedies* Sterling, New York, 1986

Reid, Daniel P. *A Handbook of Chinese Healing 'Heroes* Shambhala, Boston, 1995

Tierra, Michael *Planetary Herbology: An Integration of Western Herbs into the Traditional Chinese and Ayurvedic Systems* Lotus, Twin Lakes, 1992

Yuasa, Yasuo *The Body, Self-Cultivation, and Ki-Energy* SUNY, Albany, 1993

Zimmer, Heinrich *Hindu Medicine* Johns Hopkins University, Baltimore, 1948

CHAPTER IV: REGIONAL TRADITIONS

Ademuwagen, Z.A., A.A Ayoade, I.E. Harrison, and L. Warren (eds) *African Therapeutic Systems* Crossroads, Waltham, 1979

Ayensu, Edward S. *Medicinal Plants of West Africa* Reference, Algonac, 1978

Bastien, Joseph W. *Healers of the Andes: Kallaways Herbalists and their Medicinal Plants* University of Utan, Salt Lake City, 1987

Densmore, Francis *How Indians Use Wild Plants for Food, Medicine, and Crafts* Dover, New York, 1974

Dodge, Ernest S. *Gourd Growers of the South Seas: An Introduction to the Study of the Lagenaria Gourd in the Culture of the Polynesians* Gourd Society of America, Boston, 1943

Harjula, Raimo *Mirau and his Practice: A Study of the Ethnomedical Repertoire of a Tanzanian Herbalist* Tri-Med, London, 1980

Herrick, James W. *Iroquois Medical Botany* Syracuse University, Syracuse, 1995

Iwu, Maurice M. *Handbook of African Medicinal Plants* CRC, Boca Raton, 1993

Lebot, Vincent, Mark Merlin and Lamont Lindstrom *Kava: The Pacific Drug* Yale University, New Haven, 1992

Mooney, J. and F.M. Olbrechts "The Swimmer Manuscript: Cherokee Sacred Formulas and Medicinal Prescriptions" in *Smithsonian Institution*, Bureau of American Ethnology, Bull 99, G.P.O., Washington DC, 1932

Ngubane, Harriet *Body and Mind in Zulu Medicine* Academic, New York, 1977

Ortiz de Montellano, Bernard R. *Aztec Medicine, Health and Nutrition* Rutgers University, New Brunswick, 1990

Parsons, Claire D.F. (ed.) *Healing Practices in the South Pacific* University of Hawaii, Honolulu, 1985

Richardson, J.B. "The pre-Columbian distribution of the bottle-gourd (*Lagenaria siceraria*): a reevaluation" in *Economic Botany*, 26: 265–273, 1972

Schultes, Richard E. and Robert F. Raffauf *The Healing Forest: Medicinal and Toxic Plants of the Northwest Amazonia* Discorides, Portland, 1990

Sofowora, Abayomi *Medicinal Plants and Traditional Medicine in Africa* Wiley, New York, 1982 ·

Vogel, Virgil J. *American Indian Medicine* University of Oklahoma, Norman, 1970

Whistler, W. Arthur *Polynesian Herbal Medicine* National Tropical Botanical Garden, Lawai, Kauai, 1992

Wightman, Glen M. *Alawa Ethnobotany: Aboriginal Plant Use from Minyerri* Northern Australia Conservation Commission of the Northern Territory, Palmerston, 1991

CHAPTER V: PLANTS AND VISIONS

Anderson, Edward F. *Peyote, the Divine Cactus* University of Arizona, Tucson, 1979

Benitez, Fernando *In the Magic Land of Peyote* University of Texas, Austin, 1975

Bristol, Melvin "Tree *Datura* drugs of the Colonoian Sibundoy" in *Botanical Museum Leaflets*, 22: 165–227, Harvard University, Cambridge, 1969

Brown, Michael F. "From the hero's bones: three Aguaruna hallucinogens and their uses" in Michigan University Museum, *Anthropological Papers, No. 67: 118–136,* Ann Arbor, 1978

Fernandez, James W. *Bwiti: An Ethnography of the Religious Imagination in Africa* Princeton University, Princeton, 1982

Furst, Peter (ed.) *Flesh of the Gods: The Ritual Use of the Hallucinogens* Allen & Unwin, London, 1972

Harner, Michael H. (ed.) *Hallucinogens and Shamanism* Oxford University Press, Oxford, 1973

Hill, W.W. "Navajo use of jimsonweed" in *New Mexico Anthropologist, 3(2): 19–21,* 1938

Johnston, Thomas F. "*Datura fastuosa*: its use in Tsonga girls' initiation" in *Economic Botany 26: 340–51,* 1972; "Auditory driving, hallucinogens and music-color synesthesia in Tsonga ritual" in DuToit, B.M. (ed.) *Drugs, Rituals and Altered States of Consciousness* 217–36, Balkema, Rotterdam, 1977

Myerhoff, Barbara *Peyote Hunt: The Sacred Journey of the Huichol Indians* Cornell University, Ithaca, 1974

Ott, Jonathan *Pharmacotheon: Entheogenic Drugs, Their Plant Sources and History* Natural Products Co., Kennewick, Washington, 1993

Parsons, Elsie C. "A Zuffi detective" in *Man, 16(99): 168–70,* 1916

Petrullo, Vincenzo *The Diabolic Root* University of Pennsylvania, Philadelphia, 1934

Schleiffer, Hedwig *Sacred Narcotic Plants of the New World Indians* Hafner, New York, 1973

Schultes, Richard E. and Albert Hofmann *Plants of the Gods: Their Sacred, Healing, and Hallucinogenic Powers* McGraw-Hill, New York, 1979

Wasson, R. Gordon *The Wondrous Mushroom: Mycolotry in Mesoamerica* McGraw-Hill, New York, 1980

CHAPTER VI: HEALTH AND BEAUTY

Duff, Gail *A Book of Pot-pourri: New and Old Ideas for Fragrant Flowers and Herbs* Orbis, London, 1985

Freeman, Sally *Herbs for All Seasons: Growing and Gathering Herbs for Flavor, Health, and Beauty* Plume, New York, 1991

Genders, Roy *Natural Beauty: The Practical Guide to Wildflower Cosmetics* Webb & Bower, Exeter, 1986

Gruenberg, Louise M. *Potpourri: The Art of Fragrance Craiting* Frontier Cooperative Herbs, Norway, Iowa, 1984

Kneipp, Sebastian *My Water Cure* Health Research, Mokelumoe Hill, California, 1972

McGilvery, Carole and Jimi Reed *Essentials of Aromatherapy* Anness, London, 1994

Meyer, David *Herbal Recipes: For Hair, Salves and Liniments, Medicinal Wines and Vinegars, Plant Ash Uses* Merybooks, Glenwood, 1970

Morris, Edwin T. *Fragrance: The Story of Perfume from Cleopatra to Chanel* Scribener, New York, 1984

Tisserand, Maggie *Aromatherapy for Women: A Practical Guide to Essential Oils for Health and Beauty* Healing Arts, Rochester, 1980

Van Toller, Steven and George H. Dodd (eds) *Perfumery: The Psychology and Biology of Fragrance* Chapman and Hall, London, 1988

DOCUMENTARY REFERENCE

Altman, Nathaniel *Sacred Trees* Sierra Club, San Francisco, 1994

Bonavia, Emanuel *The Flora of the Assyrian Monuments and its Outcomes* Constable, Westminster, 1894

Caldecott, Moyra *Myths of the Sacred Tree* Destiny, Rochester, 1993

Cook, Roger *The Tree of Life* Thames & Hudson, London, 1978

Folkard, Richard *Plant Lore, Legends and Lyrics* Low, Marston, Searle & Rivington, London, 1884

Frazer, James G. *The Golden Bough* Macmillan, New York, 1974; London, 1990

Gubernatis, Angelo de *La Mythologie des Plantes; ou, Les Legendes du Regne Vegetal* Reinwald, Paris, 1882

Gupta, Shaki M. *Plant Myths and Traditions in India* Brill, Leidon, 1971

Majuparia, Trilok Chandra *Religious and Useful Plants of Nepal and India: Medicinal Plants and Flowers as Mentioned in Religious Myths and Legends of Hinduism and Buddhism* M. Gupta, Laskar, Gwalior, 1988

Parker, Arthur C. "Certain Iroquois tree myths and symbols" in *American Anthropologist, 14: 608–620,* 1912

Porteous, Alexander *Forest Folklore, Mythology, and Romance* Allen & Unwin, London, 1928

Sen Gupta, Sankar *Sacred Trees Across Cultures and Nations* Indian Publications, Calcutta, 1980

Skinner, Charles M. *Myths and Legends of Flowers, Trees, Fruits, and Plants* Lippincott, Philadelphia, 1925

Thiselton-Dyer, Thomas *The Folk-lore of Plants* Chatto & Windus, London, 1889

Useful addresses

Always send a self-addressed, stamped envelope when making an enquiry.

General Societies

The Herb Society (UK)
77 Great Peter Street
London SW1 2E

The Herb Society of America (US)
9019 Kirtland-Chardon Road
Mentor, OH44060
Tel: (216) 256 0514
(Educational herbal organization, offers a large selection of publications)

British Holistic Medical Association (UK)
179 Gloucester Place
London NW1 6DX
Tel: (0171) 262 5299
(An organization of doctors, other practitioners and non-professtionals interested in holistic medicine)

National Institute of Medical Herbalists (UK)
56 Longbrook Street
Exeter
Devon EX4 6AH
Tel: (01392) 426022

American Botanical Council (US)
P.O. Box 201660
Austin, RX 78720
Tel: (512) 331 8868
(Educational and research organization, publishes the magazine, *HerbalGram*, which covers research briefs, government rulings and herb industry news)

Herb Suppliers

Martin & Pleasance (Australia)
Wholesale Pty Ltd

P.O. Box 4
Collingwood, Victoria 3066
Tel: (6139) 419 9733

Ellon (Bach USA) Inc. (US)
P.O. Box 320
Woodmere, NY 11598
Tel: (516) 593 2206

Indiana Botanic Gardeners (US)
P.O. Box 5
Hammond, IN 46325
Tel: (219) 947 4040

Health Centre for Better Living Inc. (Italy)
6189 Tayor Road
Naples, FL 33942

Holland Pharma (Netherlands)
Postbus 37
7240 AA Lochem
Tel: (5730) 2884

Camette (Denmark)
Murerveg
6700 Esbjerg
Tel: (41) 55444

Frank Roberts (Herbal Dispensaries) Ltd (UK)
91 Newfoundland Road
Bristol BS2 9LT
Tel: (0137) 657 2456

Suffolk Herbs Ltd (UK)
Sawyer's farm
Little Conrad
Sudbury
Suffolk CO10 0NY
Tel: (0137) 657 2456

Neal's Yard Apothecary (UK)
2 Neal's Yard
London WC2
Tel: (0171) 379 7222

Aromatherapy

American Aromatherapy
Association (US)

3949 Longridge Avenue
Sherman Oaks, CA 91423
Tel: (818) 986 0594

Essential Oil Traders Association Ltd (UK)
Sarnett House
Rapton Drive
Gidea Park
Essex RM2 5LP
Tel: (0170) 820289

International Federation of Aromatherapists (UK)
Department of Continuing Education
The Royal Mesonic Hospital
Ravenscourt Park
London W6 OTN
Tel: (0181) 846 8066

Association of Aromatherapists (Australia)
693 Rathdoune Street
Carlton
Victoria
Tel: (03) 817 6431

Aroma–Therapy Supplies (UK)
52 St Aubyns Road
Fishergate
Brighton BN4 1PE
Tel: (01273) 412139

Herbalism Schools

Institute for Traditional Medicine and Preventive Health Care (US)
215 John Street
Santa Cruz, CA 95060
(Offers training programme in Chinese herbology)

National College of Naturopathic Medicine (US)
11231 S.E. Market Street
Portland, OR 97216
Tel: (503) 255 4860
(Oldest naturopathic college in the United States, awarding a Ph.D. in naturopathy)

Plant index

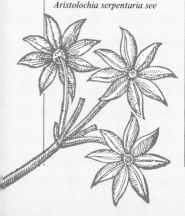

General index

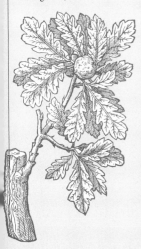

Picture credits

The publishers thank the photographers and organizations for their kind permission to reproduce the following photographs in this book:

Abbreviations
B below; **C** centre; **T** top; **L** left; **R** right
BAL The Bridgeman Art Library
FLPA Frank Lane Picture Agency
MEPL Mary Evans Picture Library
NHPA Natural History Photographic Agency
OSF Oxford Scientific Films
V&A Victoria and Albert Museum, London
WFA Werner Forman Archive

2 BAL/by courtesy of the Board of Trustees of the V&A; **7** BAL/Bibliotheque Nationale, Paris

Plants and People
8–9 Michael Freeman; **10** e.t archive; **11T** Liz Eddison/Action for Blind People; **11B** e.t. archive/Bodleian Library; **12T** Peter Gorman; **12B** NHPA; **13L** Bruce Coleman Ltd/Robert P. Carr; **13R** e.t. archive; **14L** e.t. archive; **15L** BAL/V&A **15R** e.t. Archive; **16** Bruce Coleman Ltd/Nicholas De Vore; **17T** MEPL; **17B** FLPA/Roger Wilmhurst; **18** BAL/British Library; **19T** BAL/Trinity College, Cambridge; **19B** Bruce Coleman Ltd/G. Zeisler; **20** BAL/Linnean Society; **21** e.t. archive; **22L** Edward Parker; **22R** FLPA/Eric & David Hosking; **23** e.t. archive; **24T** Bruce Coleman Ltd/David Austin; **24B** Alistair Shearer; **25** Impact Photos/Caroline Penn

Herbal Lexicon
26–7 BAL/Eton College, Windsor; **30BL** Österreichsche National Bibliothek, Vienna; **30BR** MEPL; **31B** MEPL; **32BL** MEPL; **34B** BAL/St Peter's, Leuven; **35B** BAL/Rijksmuseum Kroller-Muller, Otterlo; **36B** Bryan & Cherry Alexander; **37** Bruce Coleman Ltd/Nielsen; **38BL** Wildlife Matters; **38BR** Bruce Coleman Ltd/Hans Reinhard; **39** Hutchison Library/Christine Pemberton; **40BR** Bruce Coleman Ltd/B&C Calhoun; **41B** Art Resource/The Pierpoint Morgan Library; **42B** e.t. archive/Bodleian Library; **43B** Clive Nichols; **44B** BAL/British Museum; **45B** BAL/Giraudon; **46B** Bruce Coleman Ltd/Jane Burton; **47** BAL/Palazzo Pitti, Florence; **48R** Bruce Coleman Ltd/Dr Frieder Sauer; **49B** Wellcome Institute Library, London; **50B** BAL/Lambeth Palace Library, London; **51** BAL/Galleria Degli Offizi, Florence; **52B** Michael Holford; **53B** Austrian National Tourist Office; **56B** e.t.archive; **57B** Bruce Coleman Ltd/Michael Freeman; **58T** MEPL; **59T** OSF/Geoff Fenn; **60B** WFA **61** BAL/Lauros-Giraudon; **62B** MEPL; **63B** BAL/Bibliotheque Nationale, Paris; **65T** Bruce Coleman Ltd/Hans Reinhard; **65B** Bruce Coleman Ltd/Michael Klinec; **66B** Deni Bown; **68B** Trip/Helene Rogers; **69T** BAL/The Lindley Library; **69B** Science Photo Library

Herbal Healing in the East
72–3 Alistair Shearer; **74** Alistair Shearer; **75** The Hutchison Library; **76** Ed Stewart; **77T** Alistair Shearer; **77B** Panos Pictures/R. Berriedale-Johnson; **79T** Panos Pictures/John Miles; **79B** Alistair Shearer; **82T** Ed Stewart; **82B** Jean-Loup Charmet; **83T** MEPL; **83B** Ancient Art & Architecture Collection; **85T** Ed Stewart; **86T** WFA/Philip Goldman Collection; **86B** Agiajra/Impact Visions; **87** Ed Stewart; **90L** Robert Harding Picture Library/Robert Francis; **90R** Robert Harding Picture Library/Alain Evrard; **91T** Liz Eddison; **91B** Robert Harding Picture Library/James Strachan

Regional Traditions
92–3 Peter Furst; **94T** Ed Stewart; **94B** Bruce Coleman Ltd/Trevor Barrett; **95** Trip/C. Treppe; **96** Panos Pictures/Jeremy Hartley; **97R** Edward Parker; **98T** Ed Stewart; **98B** Art Whistler; **99T** Zefa/D. Baglin; **99B** OSF/Babs & Bertie Wells; **100** Bruce Coleman Ltd; **101T** The Harry Smith Collection; **101C** Trip/M. Ockenden; **101B** Anthrophoto/Katz; **102T** Ed Stewart; **102B** WFA/Private Collection, New York; **103T** FLPA/L. West; **103B** BAL/National Museum of American Art; **104** BAL/Royal Ontario Museum; **105T** WFA/Plains Indian Museum, Wyoming; **105B** Robert Harding Picture Library; **106L** Peter Newark's American Pictures; **106R** Peter Newark's American Pictures; **107L** Peter Furst; **107R** Deni Bown; **108** Deni Bown; **109T** WFA; **109B** OSF/Jack Dermid; **110TL** Ed Stewart; **110L** Trip/R. Powers; **110R** e.t. archive; **111** Peter Furst; **112B** Peter Furst; **112T** South American Pictures/Tony Morrison; **113** South American Pictures/Tony Morrison; **114T** Ed Stewart; **114B** Peter Furst; **115** The Hutchison Library/Edward Parker; **116L** Peter Furst; **116B** Peter Gorman; **117** S. Flores; **118T** The Hutchison Library/Eric Lawrie; **118B** The Hutchison Library/M. McIntyre; **119** The Hutchison Library

Plants and Visions
120–21 Eduardo Luna/Pablo Amarigo; **122** Peter Furst; **123** Peter Furst; **124** Peter Furst; **125T** Peter Furst; **125B** S. Flores; **126T** Peter Furst; **126B** The Hutchison Library/B. D. Drader; **127T** Peter Furst; **127B.** Harvard Botanical Library/by courtesy of Mrs Masha Arnold; **128** Peter Furst; **129** Peter Furst

Health and Beauty
130–31 e.t. archive; **132** BAL/Musée Condé, Chantilly; **133** e.t. archive; **134** Jerry Harpur/Designer: Julia Scott; **135** BAL/British Library; **137** The Anthony Blake Photo Library/James Murphy; **138** BAL/Giraudon; **154T** Robert Harding Picture Library; **154B** BAL/Louvre; **155** e.t. archive; **156** C. M. Dixon; **157T** Trip/Helene Rogers; **157B** Panos Pictures/Penny Tweedie; **158** Robert Harding Picture Library/Gerald Hoberman

Documentary Reference
160 BAL/Kunsthistorisches Museum, Vienna; **161** MEPL; **162** MEPL; **163** MEPL; **165** Dover Publications; **166** Heather Angel; **167** Peter Furst; **168** Peter Furst; **169** Peter Furst; **184** Dover Publications

Every effort has been made to trace copyright holders. However, if there are any omissions we would be happy to insert them in future editions.

Supplementary Notes
Plants work as medicines only because they can have a powerful effect upon the human body. In addition, some healing plants look very similar to other, poisonous, plants. Never use a plant unless it is prescribed by a qualified herbalist or unless you are absolutely sure of its botanical identity, its safety and how to use it. The information contained in this book is introductory in nature and is not intended as a substitute for professional knowledge. Neither the publishers nor the author can accept any responsibility for the unsafe use of plants by readers.

The cultivation and harvesting times given in this book are for temperate Europe and North America, where the average last frost is at the end of April and the average first frost is at the end of October. Readers in other parts of the world should adjust the times accordingly.

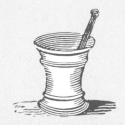